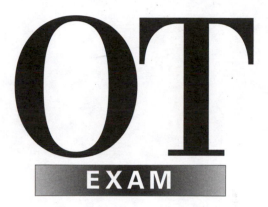

REVIEW MANUAL

FOURTH EDITION

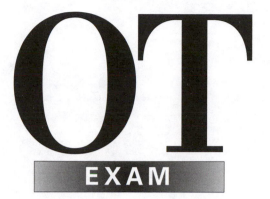

REVIEW MANUAL

FOURTH EDITION

Karen Sladyk, PhD, OTR/L, FAOTA
Bay Path College
Longmeadow, Massachusetts

with

Signian McGeary, MS, OTR/L
Quinnipiac University
Hamden, Connecticut

Lori S. Gilmore, MS, CSE
Rockville High School
Vernon, Connecticut

Roseanna Tufano, MFT, OTR/L
Quinnipiac University
Hamden, Connecticut

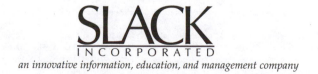

SLACK
INCORPORATED
an innovative information, education, and management company

6900 Grove Road • Thorofare, NJ 08086

OT exam review manual / Karen Sladyk ; with Signian McGeary, Lori S. Gilmore, Roseanna Tufano.-- 4th ed.
    p. ; cm.
Includes bibliographical references and index.
ISBN 1-55642-702-6 (alk. paper)
1. · Occupational therapy--Examinations, questions, etc. 2. Occupational therapy--Outlines, syllabi, etc.
[DNLM: 1. Occupational Therapy--Examination Questions. WB 18.2 O88 2005] I. Title: Occupational therapy exam review manual. II. Sladyk, Karen, 1958- III. Title.

RM735.32.O87 2005
615.8'515'076--dc22   2004018795

Published by: SLACK Incorporated
                     6900 Grove Road
                     Thorofare, NJ 08086 USA
                     Telephone: 856-848-1000
                     Fax: 856-853-5991
                     www.slackbooks.com

Contact SLACK Incorporated for more information about other books in this field or about the availability of our books from distributors outside the United States.

Authorization to photocopy items for internal or personal use, or the internal or personal use of specific clients, is granted by SLACK Incorporated, provided that the appropriate fee is paid directly to Copyright Clearance Center, 222 Rosewood Drive, Danvers, MA 01923 USA, 978-750-8400. Prior to photocopying items for educational classroom use, please contact the CCC at the address above. Please reference Account Number 9106324 for SLACK Incorporated's Professional Book Division.

For further information on CCC, check CCC Online at the following address: http://www.copyright.com.

Last digit is print number: 10 9 8 7 6 5 4 3 2 1

DEDICATION

To every occupational therapy student and the teachers
and clinicians who educate them.

CONTENTS

ACKNOWLEDGMENTS

No book would be complete without thanking all the people behind the scenes. This is true for all of us as well. Lori G., Roseanna, Signian, Julie, Lori V., and I want to thank our families for their support. A special thank you to our friends at SLACK Incorporated, especially Amy McShane, Debra Toulson, Lauren Plummer, and Jennifer Cahill. My friends from the University of Connecticut, Department of Adult and Vocational Education, deserve special thanks for their "of course you can do that" attitude. Many former OT students, now OTs, were helpful in the development of this book, including Erika Lund, Wendy Carpenter, Pam Guyette, Rory Marcello, and Jeff Abrahamson. The second edition also contained several review questions written by Christine Negro, OT student. We are especially pleased that a student who has not even begun to study for the exam was able to write such dynamic questions. The third edition was reviewed by the first graduating OT class of Bay Path College, Longmeadow, MA, and the fourth edition adds another student voice, that of Lori Vaughn, now an OT. Lastly, a special thank you to all occupational therapy students, past, present, and future, for reminding us what teaching is all about. May this book bring you great success on the exam and may your healing hands touch many hearts and minds.

ABOUT THE AUTHORS

Karen Sladyk, PhD, OTR/L, FAOTA, has a BS in Occupational Therapy from Eastern Michigan University, Ypsilanti; an MS in Community Health from Southern Connecticut State University, New Haven; and a PhD in Adult and Vocational Education from the University of Connecticut, Storrs. Karen teaches at Bay Path College in Longmeadow, MA. Her occupational therapy interests include clinical reasoning and fieldwork. She resides in Tolland, CT in a small house with two cats. When she is not busy with academic challenges, she enjoys quilt making.

Signian McGeary, MS, OTR/L, has 25 years of adult physical disability practice following her degree in Occupational Therapy from Quinnipiac University, Hamden, CT. Her transition into teaching has resulted in a MS in Adult Education. Her current clinical interests include a research study in hip fractures and international travel. She has studied Mandarin Chinese to prepare for educational clinical exchanges in China with the World Health Organization. She has taken students to numerous countries for nontraditional fieldwork and will teach OT in Africa next year. Her husband, two daughters, and son-in-law, as well as her grandchildren, share and support her love of international travel.

Lori S. Gilmore, MS, CSE, has a BS degree in Social Work from Southern Connecticut State University, New Haven; a teaching certificate in Special Education; and a MS in Language Arts from Central Connecticut State College, New Britain. She has completed an advanced graduate degree in Learning Disabilities at the University of Connecticut, Storrs. When she is not busy with work and school, she is active in community activities with her new family, including her three sons, Brent, Seth, and Blake. Lori also holds a teaching position (secondary) and enjoys quilt making but is much different from her sister, Karen Sladyk, in that she only has one cat.

Roseanna Tufano, MFT, OTR/L, has a BS degree in Occupational Therapy from Quinnipiac University, Hamden, CT. She has worked in a variety of psychiatric settings since 1980 as a staff OT and consultant. She is presently assistant professor at Quinnipiac University where she teaches psychopathology, group dynamics, clinical media, and psychosocial aspects of physical disabilities. Roseanna completed her master's in Marriage and Family Therapy. She resides with her husband, Lou, and their two children, Carissa and Brett. They continue to be her source for love, inspiration, and fun.

PREFACE

Becoming an OT is not a simple task. Getting into an occupational therapy program, completing the schooling, the months of fieldwork, and finally the certification exam takes a lot of time, commitment, and effort. Many of us who are OTs think occupational therapy is the best career you could choose even in these changing times. This study guide is designed to help you get ready for the last step in becoming an OT—the certification exam.

This study guide is designed with the student in mind. It is lovingly written by experts in the field of occupational therapy with the sole purpose of helping you get through the studying process and successfully negotiating the certification exam. Although the material is serious, we have attempted to make it light and humorous when possible. To make it easier to read, we have provided the information you need in paragraphs with clear headings.

The book is divided into four main sections: Getting Ready, Study Techniques, Study Questions, and Life After the Exam. The first section deals with a general overview of the examination process. Also included are numerous tools to get yourself organized. The second section includes chapters on content and using your fieldwork experiences to guide your studying. The third section contains 600 study questions set up in the same format as the certification exam. The certification exam is made up of 200 questions with a 4-hour time limit, so our study questions are divided into groups of 50 with a time limit of 1 hour. The last section deals with life after the exam and provides some practical advice if things do not go well. New to this edition is a web site to practice reading questions on a computer screen. Although not a "practice exam," this web site can provide valuable information to your study program.

We have also included information in the appendices you might find helpful. In Appendix C, you will find a feedback sheet for us. After you have studied for the exam, we would appreciate a short note from you about this book. Let us know what you liked and did not like about the book. Is there something you wished we had done differently? Future students will benefit from your insights.

Best wishes,

Karen Sladyk, PhD, OTR/L, FAOTA

SECTION 1
Getting Ready

Chapter One

Overview

Karen Sladyk, PhD, OTR/L, FAOTA, and Lori Vaughn, OTR/L

WHAT TO DO FIRST

Many students preparing for the OT exam ask the question "What should I do first?" The answer is "It depends." This study guide includes information for every type of person. Where you start depends on how much time you have left to study. In an attempt to give you some structure, let's first look at how much time you have between opening this book for the first time and the certification exam. Calculate the time you have until the next exam, then check the table below for a suggestion of what to do next.

Assuming you have at least 40 hours of study time ahead of you, the entire study guide is within reach. A good place to start is right here. A little history about the certification process will give you a better understanding of the exam.

WHAT TO DO FIRST

Time Left Until the Next Exam	Start Your Reading Here
6 or more months	Good for you, you have plenty of time to study. Read the entire study guide. Study 1 to 2 hours per week. Use the web site when ready.
4 to 5 months	You planned well. Read the entire study guide. Begin with 3 to 4 hours per week. Use the web site when ready.
2 to 3 months	No need to panic. You have some time, but you must be efficient. Read the entire study guide this week. Aim for an hour per day until the study guide is completed. Adjust your study time from there. Use the web site when ready.
About 1 month	Time to get serious. Read the entire study guide this week. Aim for at least 1 to 2 hours per day until the study guide is completed. Begin your study plan developed in Chapter Two. Use the web site when ready.
3 weeks	Skip Chapters One and Seven for now. Begin with Chapters Two and Five. Try at least 100 questions in Chapter Five and 50 questions from Chapter Six or the web site. Adjust your study plan from there.
2 weeks	Complete Chapter Six or the web site. Read Chapters Two and Four. Develop a study plan from there.

WHAT TO DO FIRST (CONTINUED)

Time Left Until the Next Exam	*Start Your Reading Here*
1 week or less	Complete Chapter Six or the web site. Skim Chapters Two and Four for test-taking suggestions.
If you are already an OT and are using this book for review	If you are taking the exam: Begin with Chapters Five and Six. Skim Chapters Two and Four. If you are not taking the exam but doing a review: Complete Chapters Five and Six.

CERTIFICATION PROCESS

The National Board for Certification in Occupational Therapy (NBCOT) is a private, nonprofit agency responsible for the development and administration of the certification exam for OTs. In addition, NBCOT manages the exam for certification of OTAs. Management of each exam requires development of high standards to protect and serve the public. This ensures quality occupational therapy personnel are entering the profession. NBCOT meets the challenge by developing policies and working closely with the development committee with test and measurement experts to ensure quality. Although certification of an OT may not be required by a few work sites, most governmental, regulatory, insurance, and other agencies use NBCOT examinations as a credential standard. Many state licensing boards require passing the certification exam as the minimum standard for employment.

OT Examination Question Development

The questions on the OT certification exam are based on a survey conducted of practicing OTs and educators to establish the knowledge of entry-level clinicians. The study focused on the skills needed by a new graduate to successfully practice occupational therapy. The study results are used by the Certification Examination Development Committee (CEDC) to develop new exam questions. Expert OTs from a variety of work settings across the country make up the NBCOT CEDC. The 14 members of this committee are trained in item writing and develop exam questions specific to their content area. All items are rigorously reviewed by the CEDC before appearing as examination questions. Item writers use the American Occupational Therapy Association (AOTA) document *The Occupational Therapy Practice Framework* as a basis for terminology. This publication is available in the *American Journal of Occupational Therapy,* November/December 2002, or by calling AOTA at 301-652-2682 (1-800-SAY-AOTA if you are a student member).

OT Examination Administration

The NBCOT contracts with a professional testing company to ensure high standards of reliability and validity in the test development and administration. The professional testing agency is responsible for administering and scoring the exam as well as reporting the results to the student. Each OT certification exam is a unique combination of exam items pulled from a data bank of possible questions. The data banks for OTAs and OTs are kept separate, and the questions are never used in both exams. NBCOT provides a list of content areas and the percentage of weight for each area to the test taker prior to the exam. This outline ensures consistency between the tests over time.

Application for the OT Examination

The program director at your school will provide you with information on how to begin the application process for the NBCOT exam. Additional information can be found on NBCOT's website at www.nbcot.org. Download a candidate's handbook at the appropriate time for taking your exam and follow the directions carefully, including the policies for fees. Failure to follow the rules will result in denial of your application. Online registration is the most common and preferred method because the computer will tell you if you have left any blanks on the application. In addition, computer application is less expensive.

OT Examination Structure

Each exam has 200 multiple choice questions. Each question will have four possible choices labeled A through D. There are no "all of the above" or combination choices on the OT exam. The penalty for leaving an answer blank is the same as an incorrect answer, so be sure to complete your best guess for all items. Choose only one answer for each question, and key in the correct answer on the computer. The examination will be scored by the testing agency and then reviewed by the CEDC to look for flawed questions.

After flawed questions are removed, criterion-referenced scoring will be used to calculate the passing score. This means that those people above the criterion score will pass the certification examination and those below will not.

Your score is not compared to other people who took the exam, but simply compared to the minimum passing level to be an entry-level occupational therapist. Test takers who need special accommodations due to a disability (e.g., visual, hearing, health, or orthopedic impairment; or learning, emotional, or multiple disabilities) will be provided with services as outlined in the Americans with Disabilities Act. Information on special accommodations is located in the candidate's handbook from NBCOT. It is important that you provide the necessary documentation and follow the specific process in the handbook.

THE "NEW" NBCOT EXAM

In March 2000, NBCOT developed a new style of certification exam. The current test reflects the professional practice survey completed in 2003. This section of the book will look at the facts about the "new" exam.

Much of the new exam structure remains unchanged. The exam still consists of 200 multiple choice questions with four possible answers. The candidates still have 4 hours to answer their questions. The questions are still entry-level occupational therapy practice questions from a variety of practice areas. So what's the new difference? The difference is how the questions are developed and classified.

Domain, Tasks, and Knowledge

The most recent practice analysis survey looked at what OTs need to know to practice occupational therapy. NBCOT developed a new blueprint in 2004 based on the practice analysis of 2003. The new structure of the exam is based on three components of a new practitioner's work: domains, tasks, and knowledge. Although no major changes were the result of this new blueprint, NBCOT has used new language that better fits with what the practice setting is using. Under NBCOT's 2004 blueprint, *domains* include:

- Evaluation
- Developing treatment plans
- Implementing meaningful treatment approaches
- Addressing population needs
- Managing OT services

Domains continue to be the foundation of the exam, and implementing meaningful interventions continues to be the area of heaviest test questions. *Tasks* are described as what practitioners do, and *knowledge* is defined as what practitioners need to know to perform tasks. Under the old blueprint, these two areas were described as content. So why is this language change so important to the person studying for the exam? Because it reinforces that your study approach must be holistic and not just focused on treatment from a pathology point of view. That said, you must also have a firm knowledge base of foundations, pathology, and management issues. The blueprint is just that, a plan or guide for NBCOT to outline questions that are as diverse as the practice of occupational therapy.

Using the domain, task, and knowledge blueprint, consider the following case:

A person with a vestibular disorder of disequilibrium due to aging is referred to occupational therapy. She is complaining that balance problems interfere with her activities.

For domain issues, you must think about evaluation, treatment, and issues of importance to this population. For task issues, you must think about what OT practitioners do with clients such as this. For knowledge issues, you must think about pathology and foundations of meaningful activities. Note how tasks and knowledge help form the domain and how the three catagories are all interlinked. This is the holistic nature of the exam questions.

Knowledge needed for the specific case of vestibular disorder of disequilibrium due to aging includes:
- There is likely loss of cells in the peripheral labyrinth as well as the central nervous system
- This likely developed over time
- There is likely loss of sensation in the foot, perhaps diabetes
- There is likely proprioception issues

Tasks common for this specific case of vestibular disorder of disequilibrium due to aging includes:
- Activities must be graded
- Transfers from sitting to standing is likely an issue, especially the bathtub
- Patient education

A domain-based question that utilizes knowledge and tasks would look like this:

A person with a vestibular disorder of disequilibrium due to aging is referred to occupational therapy. She is complaining that balance interferes with her socializing even in her house because she cannot wash and dress herself. What is the *first* issue for the OT to address?

- A. Finding ways for her to socialize using the phone
- B. Addressing safety in the bathtub
- C. Improving balance during dressing
- D. Developing a graded exercise program to improve balance

The best answer is B. All the options, finding activities that are meaningful to this client, are appropriate treatment but the first issue is always safety. As a person with this condition may have sensation issues, especially if diabetes is present, bathtub mobility becomes a safety issue immediately.

There are no questions on the NBCOT exam that ask task or knowledge questions. An example of a task questions would be: How do OTs adapt a bathroom? An example of a knowledge question would be: What inner ear cells are likely lost in aging? Since this type of question is never asked on the NBCOT exam, why include these in this study manual?

Mixed Domain, Task, and Knowledge Questions as Study Questions

This exam manual uses all three types of questions as a way to prepare you for the NBCOT exam. The questions in this book are designed as study tools, not real practice questions. On a rare occasion, we received feedback that our questions "were not like the real test." This test taker was right, these questions are designed to help you study all the material necessary to be confident in your answers on the NBCOT exam. Simply practicing real questions will only give you a pass/fail score, not prepare you to think about the questions. This goes back to the earlier comment about preparing for the NBCOT from a holistic approach including using a variety of study ideas.

When Two Sources Disagree

A student wrote us once asking for our opinion about a specific question in which our information disagreed with the information that had been presented to her by another resource. We were happy to comment on this because, in an exciting and always changing profession like occupational therapy, there are times when different professionals disagree about an issue. Our questions are study questions, designed to help you study for the exam. Because the questions are not exam questions, you may find a question in which the answer disagrees with something you learned somewhere else. In the NBCOT exam, numerous people review each question. Remember that NBCOT also removes any question from the exam after it has been administered if the question is found to be faulty.

STUDYING IDEAS

Now that you understand NBCOT and the certification process, it is time to begin making your study plan. Chapter Two of this book covers your personal study plan in great detail; however, let us briefly look at some ideas you may find helpful.

Study groups: Studying a large amount of material with a group of people can be easier and more efficient. However, not all study groups are effective. You may have experienced a group project in school in which one or more participants did not do their fair share. This often leads to resentment and hurt feelings. If you plan to form a study group, ask people you are *certain* will actively participate. If you are asked to join a study group, be sure you have a clear understanding of the group's goals and expectations. In any case, be sure to allow some time at the beginning of the first session to allow everyone an opportunity to share goals and expectations. If someone feels he or she cannot participate, allow the student to decline with dignity.

Exam review conferences: Many occupational therapy schools offer a 1- or 2-day conference to review for the exam. You can email AOTA if you are a member or an area occupational therapy school to see if one is available.

Lecture notes: Even though you may have had one class that you did not like, the faculty at your school have provided you with a global education in occupational therapy. AOTA requires all occupational therapy programs to meet minimum standards to receive or maintain the school's accreditation. Your occupational therapy program has met the essential components. This means that your classes provided you with at least the minimum information needed to pass the exam and become a practicing OT. As a result, you should have everything you need to know about occupational therapy written down in your class lecture notes. Reviewing your notes is one of the most effective ways to study for the certification exam.

Textbooks: It would be impossible (and we do not recommend) for you to reread your textbooks from cover to cover. Even if you did not sell them back to the bookstore, reading your textbooks in their entirety is not an effective use of study time.

It is appropriate to read your textbooks in the areas in which you are weak. We recommend that you read only the textbook sections in which you need a detailed review. Use your notes from class to provide a basic study outline and refer to the textbooks for more detail. Be sure to save your textbooks for your professional needs after the exam.

NBCOT practice test: NBCOT offers a practice test given by computer. This test is made up of sample questions scored by the computer, and a summary score is provided. See the candidate's handbook for fees and application processes.

We would also like to call your attention to the appendices of this book. We have provided information that you may find helpful as you study for the exam. In Appendix A, you will find a list of suggested occupational therapy references. Do not worry if you have never had a particular textbook in your classes. The suggestions are comprehensive to provide broad coverage of the material on the exam; however, your faculty has chosen an excellent blend of textbooks for you. In addition to the reference list, we have provided a list of abbreviations in Appendix B that you may find helpful. All of this information is designed to help you get ready for the "big day."

Exam Day

The day of the exam will be filled with much nervous energy. It is best to plan ahead to enhance the chances of a smooth day. The old advice of a good night's sleep and eating well before any test is especially true for taking the exam. You may want to try a dry run to the test site prior to exam day if you are unfamiliar with the location. If you are traveling on exam day and might encounter bad weather, listen to the weather report and allow extra time to get to the exam site if needed. If you are driving, fill your gas tank the day before the exam.

Wear comfortable clothes but keep in mind the season and weather. Layered clothing will allow you to adjust your clothing if the room is too warm or cool. If your hair is long, tie it back but avoid wearing a baseball cap or any other type of hat that blocks your face from the exam proctors.

Have a bag ready to take with you as you leave for the test site. Include the following items in your bag:

1. A map to the test site if you are unfamiliar with the location
2. A cell phone or change for a pay phone to call for directions or help if needed
3. A watch
4. Photo identification
5. Tissues are available at the site, however, you may bring your own earplugs
6. A snack high in complex carbohydrates (e.g., a whole-grain bagel) for long-term thinking power (eat before entering the testing room, as food is not allowed during the exam)
7. Chewing gum, if needed
8. Reading glasses, if you use them
9. Your admission paperwork
10. A pencil if you want to use scratch paper

Once you arrive at the test site, register at the front desk. While waiting to enter the exam room you may want to use the restroom. If you are anxious, avoid talking to people who will make you feel more nervous. Find a quiet space to relax. Do not study or review notes. This is the time to focus on relaxing.

A New OT's Voice

In this edition of the book, the authors have asked new OT Lori Vaughn to share her experiences with you. We are very pleased she agreed and believe her insightful comments will motivate the reader.

From the Desk of Lori Vaughn, OTR/L

In occupational therapy, there is nothing more exhilarating, or terrifying, than completing the academic requirements and fieldwork affiliations and walking toward the podium to accept your diploma at graduation. Exhilarating because you are taking the first steps toward the rest of your life. Terrifying because you are taking the first steps toward the rest of your life. Before the calligrapher's ink has dried on your diploma, the realization hits that the journey is only half over, and you must now prepare for the NBCOT registration exam.

Undertaking preparations to study is no easy task. The volumes of information that you accumulated while in school and during fieldwork can seem like an incredible, insurmountable mountain. Each day you avoid the mountain, which in actuality is the closed door behind which you have hidden all of your school "stuff." Perhaps you are hoping it will go away, thinking if you don't look at it, it doesn't exist. Or, maybe you just cannot get over that nausea that you feel every time you think about taking the exam. "I just need a break," I would tell myself. "I'm not ready yet" was another excuse. I was just overwhelmed.

One day I received an information letter regarding repayment of my student loans. This was like my wake-up call, and I realized that I could no longer continue with my excuses. My future was coming whether I was ready or not. I knew that there was only one way for me to buckle down, and that was to bite the bullet and schedule a date for the exam.

Once I had a date scheduled, I became like a woman possessed. Typically, I am an organization freak (I have been called the queen of color coding), which I believe was ultimately the key to my success. Everyone has his or her own study strategies, and the ones I describe may not be for everyone, but they worked for me. First, I bravely repeated the phrase that became my mantra throughout this experience—"You can do it… You can do it…"—and opened that dreaded door separating me from the rest of my life. I began organizing the class notes and information that were beginning to gather dust, much like my brain. As the piles of information grew, I began to internalize that phrase and think, "Yes, maybe I can do this." Next, I considered the experiences that I had during my various fieldwork affiliations. Allow me an aside here to get on my soapbox and offer my opinion regarding fieldwork. It is imperative that you make the most of every minute and take advantage of the professionals around you. Through fieldwork, you are able to hone your clinical reasoning skills, receive constructive feedback, and begin to grow as a professional. Clinical reasoning is the foundation upon which the certification exam is built, so work with your supervisors and other staff to develop these skills. My feeling with school, fieldwork, and basically every aspect of life is that you get out of it what you put in, so make the most of every moment. This will help you beyond measure to succeed, both in the exam room and in practice. That being my mindset, I then used my fieldwork experiences to supplement the information within the various categories I had created.

The next step for me involved gathering as much information as I could about the test itself. Knowing the composition of the categories and weight that each section held guided me in determining which areas I needed to further supplement. I did this through the NBCOT website, along with a variety of different study guides. The value of the study guides, such as the previous edition of this text, was immeasurable in preparing for the exam. I understood that these study guides were not "real" tests, but were designed to help me think about questions. I began taking the exams offered in the books right away. I only completed a portion of each exam at a time, so that I did not become overwhelmed with the information. That helped me to know in which areas I had a solid grasp, and in which areas I should focus more attention. Taking that first study exam was a brave and harrowing experience. Realizing how much or how little I recalled in specific areas was an eye opener, but it provided me with a plan of attack. I decided that I needed to further supplement my areas of weakness by gathering additional information from textbooks and professional websites. The piles were increasing, but so were my knowledge base and my confidence. Once I had gathered all of the information, I fell back on the skills that helped me throughout school: I planned. I purchased a large desk-sized calendar. On each day, I wrote the categories or material that I wanted to get through that day. I wrote the topics in pen, because I knew that pencil would be too easy to erase and put off until a later date. The structure is what made me successful. I mixed up the information that I really needed to focus on with the information that I already had a handle on so that if I fell behind one day, I could easily catch up the next. I then used a thick, black, permanent marker to cross out each area that I completed. There are few things as good as the sense of accomplishment and confidence you feel as the black marks begin to predominate the calendar.

I completed one-half of a study exam each week. Most guides provide rationale for correct answers, together with outlining why the other options were incorrect. I completed the pencil and paper tests so that I could look back at them as part of my studying. Many of the books provide disks, which are helpful in providing a testing experience more similar to the actual exam. I am a concrete person, so being able to refer back to the paper exam was the most effective for me.

Another strategy I used was to go online and read postings and messages from other people who had taken the exam. One day when I was looking for information on the exam, I typed in NBCOT into the search engine. What I found was a network of people, much like myself, who were about to take the exam or had recently received their results. This was very affirming because it let me know that I was not alone and, pass or fail, I would not be the first, or the last, to do either. I also found success stories, much like the one I am now able to write, with advice, opinions, and lists of useful resources. This was an extremely valuable tool that I had no idea existed. It was like a secret society of OT students. There was no secret handshake, but the camaraderie that developed between people who have shared the same pleasure, and pain, was invaluable. This is where I get on my soapbox again. As students, we live two lives—one with our home families and one with our school families. Both of these are essential to your success. I will not expound upon the value of a good base of support at home. I think that that is well documented. However, I will tout the importance of your school family. Only an OT student knows what it is like to be an OT student. No one else has walked in those shoes, no matter what other professional degrees he or she may hold. Use that bond to work together to plan, study, or share materials, or to vent to someone who knows.

When my exam date was approximately 6 weeks away, I began taking the NBCOT practice exams online. There is a fee for these, however for me, it was money well spent. These exams are comprised of 100 questions, are timed, and are set up in a similar fashion to the actual exam, with the same percentage of questions in each domain as appear on the full exam. You receive the results right away, with an outline of your performance in each of the domains. The only negative aspect is that there is no breakdown of correct and incorrect responses, so you do not know which questions you answered correctly, nor do you receive a rationale for specific answers. This is a reason why it is important to use a variety of sources.

NBCOT permits a person to take three online practice exams, so I spread these out over the next few weeks. I saved the last one for the week before my scheduled exam, figuring it would give me a confidence boost if I did well, or outline the final area(s) that still needed attention if I did poorly. Luckily, it was the former rather than the latter, which put a small dent in the growing anxiety as the date approached. Ultimately, the score that I achieved on each of the three practice exams was almost identical to that which I scored on the actual exam.

When I scheduled my exam, I decided to schedule it for a Tuesday. That was a conscious decision. I figured that I could have the weekend to lock myself behind that previously closed door, within the room in which my presence amongst the piles of school "stuff" had become commonplace over the past several weeks. I thought I could then take Monday to relax and recuperate in preparation for the big day. Of course, this was wishful thinking. At that point, it is difficult to shut down because all you can think about is absorbing as much information as you can. In hindsight, I should have stuck with the original plan. What I had not learned up to that day would not have made as much a difference as a good night's sleep might have made. Knowing my personal study habits, however, I needed to take advantage of each minute to study in order to feel comfortable. Also, knowing that I am more of a morning person, I decided to schedule the exam first thing in the morning. It is important to have a good sense of yourself when making exam preparations in order to achieve the best outcome.

Some important things to consider when scheduling the exam are the location of the testing center, the time of day you want to take it, and the route you will take to get there. If you are unfamiliar with the area, take a trial run on the same day of the week and time that you have scheduled the exam so that you can get a sense of how much traffic there will be on that day and how much time it will take to get there. Then, add an extra 20 to 30 minutes just in case of an emergency. There is nothing worse than having something unforeseen happen, and then have to rush to get to the testing center. There is enough stress related to taking the exam under ideal circumstances.

Also, although your stomach may feel like it is auditioning for the Olympic tumbling team, try to eat something. The author of this study guide offered me some words of wisdom in that regard. Try to eat some carbohydrates (sorry Atkins fans). You are like an athlete running a 4-hour marathon, and you want to make sure that you have enough energy to reach the finish line. Also, try to get that rest that I mentioned. You want to give your brain and body time to oxygenate and rejuvenate. Having a clear and focused mind is essential.

As you drive, listen to your favorite CD or radio station. This will give your mind a break. Some people prefer quiet during the ride, but I found that this made my mind wander into areas of uncertainty, and that is the last thing that I wanted in my head before the exam. In addition, when you arrive at the testing center, try not to take the closest parking space. Find a spot that will require a little walking. We all know the value of exercise in allowing the nervous system to calm and organize. As you walk, take some deep breaths and really draw the oxygen into your lungs. Your body and brain will thank you. Extra materials are not permitted into the testing area, but leave yourself a treat in the car. Chocolate works great for this! You will need something comforting once you are finished, and you should be rewarded for all of your hard work.

My testing center provided both earplugs and headphones for the exam. All provide one or the other, if not both. Use at least one of them. It will allow you to concentrate and not be distracted by any sounds that are around you. Also, try not to consume too much liquid before the exam. You are permitted to go to the restroom, but your time continues to run. If you are typically a coffee drinker, make sure you have at least a small cup, otherwise you may end up with a caffeine withdrawal headache.

As you are taking the exam, go through and answer as many questions as you can. Mark the ones that you are not sure of or just want to go back and recheck. Be sure to read each question carefully. Sometimes the question asks for the *most* likely answer, and sometimes it asks for the *least* likely. Take your time and read every word. Also, pay some attention to the clock, but do not become obsessed by the time. It is good to be aware of where you stand, but you cannot let it distract you. I found it helpful to plan to average about 1 minute per question. That left me approximately 40 minutes to go back and check the questions I marked. Some questions took much less than 1 minute, but some took more.

When you finish the exam, it is important to not start second-guessing yourself. Go back to the car and enjoy your special treat. Whether you have left yourself that chocolate, or something healthier, such as a new CD, savor every minute and try not to dwell on the questions. This is easier said than done, because the only questions that will be running through your mind are the ones that you are not sure you answered correctly. For me, the ones that I found easy were long forgotten, and all that I could think about were the ones that I found more difficult. This led me to convince myself that I had failed. I began making contingency plans for when I received the inevitable results. The only thing on my mind was what I would do when, not if, I failed. I tried to put my mind on other things, but it invariably came back to the test. Although I questioned several of my responses, I avoided opening a single textbook or looking at any of my notes. To me, the uncertainty was better than the possibility of confirming that I had answered questions incorrectly.

Each day that passes while awaiting the test results is like an eternity. You find yourself completing busy work just to occupy your mind. It is a good idea to plan something fun for this time, such as a vacation or day trips. Any distraction is a blessing. For me, my friends and family tried to provide the moral support that I intrinsically lacked. I was showered with their confidence in me, but it really did little to help. How could they be so confident, when I was not? I write this not to cause any additional fear or reservation to that which you may already be experiencing, but to let you know that post-test anxiety is normal and something that each of us who has been there has experienced. After you take the exam, I recommend rereading these pages. There is comfort in knowing that what you are feeling is typical and that each of us has experienced the same emotions.

The day that the results arrived could not come too quickly for me, but even when it did, I was not quite ready. The culmination of all of the years of school and months of studying rested in my very shaky hands. There is nothing that prepares you for the roller coaster of emotions that you experience at that very moment. You engage in a sublime conversation with yourself deciding whether or not to open the letter. The minutes tick by, but you are not aware of their passage, transfixed only on the envelope until the need to know finally overtakes you.

The anxiety that made my hands tremble was quickly replaced by exuberance as I read the paper that began with "Congratulations…" There is little to compare to the feeling of elation upon reading that single word. Being on the threshold of a career path that I love has made every second of work worthwhile. It has been said that anything worth having is worth working for, and this is no exception. It is a tremendous task that is ahead of you as you begin this process, but remember that success is within your grasp and your future is an open door.

COUNTDOWN CALENDAR

A blank calendar is provided to help you organize your last month before the exam. Use this calendar to chart your goals and study plans. Begin by entering the month and year you will take the exam. Enter the dates in each box. Enter the exam date and fill in the other dates on the calendar. Remove the calendar from the book and post it in a prominent place. Once you have a dated calendar of your goals, you can begin to develop your study plans in Chapter Two.

SUMMARY

Beginning to study for the certification exam can be overwhelming. Information on where to start is provided in this chapter. The role of NBCOT and the history and process of the exam are reviewed to help you understand the exam. General study techniques and a countdown calendar are provided to guide you through your exam preparation. Information for a smooth exam day is also included.

COUNTDOWN CALENDAR						
Sunday	*Monday*	*Tuesday*	*Wednesday*	*Thursday*	*Friday*	*Saturday*

Section II
Study Techniques

Chapter Two

How to Study for the Exam

GETTING STARTED

Congratulations! Obviously you care enough about your upcoming exam to purchase and read this book. Okay, so you couldn't part with the money, but you asked your parents to buy it for you. Even if you *borrowed* this book, your intentions are still good. You've done well enough in college to get to this point. You don't need a "how to" study guide because you have already been successful. However, you may wish to look at your current study habits and determine whether you can be a more efficient learner. Perhaps there is a study technique that you have not thought of or a memory strategy that can benefit you. The purpose of this chapter is to help you select the study techniques that will benefit you.

You are in charge. No one will know if you are in your room studying or reading a magazine. You are responsible for your study plan. Studying may be a burden, but it is a light one to bear considering the alternatives: having fun, going out, watching TV, etc. Oh all right! There are other things you could be doing, but you may not get the same result. Effective studying will give you satisfaction, peace of mind, and added confidence. You will know that no matter what the outcome, you have done your best and can hold your head high.

Remember, you are a unique individual. Do not waste time comparing yourself to others studying for the exam. Your experiences and personal situations are different than others'. Accept your personal strengths and weaknesses, and develop a plan of attack based on your needs. Listen to others' good suggestions but stick to the plan that will benefit you. Be honest in your own assessments and be willing to admit if something is not working. Evaluate your plan regularly to see if you are obtaining the results you intended. If not, modify your plan based on what you need.

Take the time now to make a plan. Even if it is a lousy one, you are heading in the right direction. You can always change it later, but at least relieve some stress by making some decisions. The following pages will assist you in assessing your current learning preferences in order to develop an effective plan.

FINDING YOUR BEST LEARNING STYLE

Learning styles refer to the way people take in, store, and retrieve information. Some people learn and remember best by hearing, while others learn by writing. You may have a preference for one style or modality, or you may find that a combination of styles works best for you. Take the following inventory to help determine your strongest learning preference. Check the following characteristics that apply to you.

LEARNING STYLE CHARACTERISTICS CHECKLIST

1. ___When I have a problem, I usually tell someone right away.
2. ___I keep a journal.
3. ___I often take notes, although I do not always refer to them.
4. ___I take good notes, then rewrite them at a later time.
5. ___I read in my free time.
6. ___I have the TV on even if I am not watching it.

7. ___I have good intentions of writing to people but usually call instead.
8. ___I often shut my eyes to help myself concentrate.
9. ___When studying or solving a problem, I pace back and forth.
10. ___I would rather hear a book on audiocassette than read it myself.
11. ___Forget the cassette, I would rather wait until it comes out on film.
12. ___I prefer reading the newspaper to watching the news on TV.
13. ___I prefer to study in a quiet setting.
14. ___To remember a spelling, I "see" the word in my mind.
15. ___I would prefer an oral exam to a written one.
16. ___I prefer a multiple choice format on a test.
17. ___I would rather do a project than write a paper.
18. ___I would rather give an oral report than a written one.
19. ___I remember better what I read rather than what I hear.
20. ___I keep a personal organizer.
21. ___I reread my notes several times.
22. ___I would rather take notes from the text than attend a lecture on the material.
23. ___I often "talk to myself."
24. ___I learn best when I study with a partner.
25. ___I can locate a passage that I have read by "seeing it."
26. ___I find it hard to sit still when I study.
27. ___If I forgot why I walked into the kitchen, I retrace my steps from the bedroom.
28. ___Once in bed for the night, I shut my eyes and plan the next day.
29. ___I cannot clean unless the music is on.
30. ___I would rather read directions than have someone tell me about them.
31. ___I can put something together as long as the directions are written.

SCORING THE CHECKLIST

Compare your answers from your checklist to the checklist below. Circle the letters that correspond to your answers.

1. **S**   When I have a problem, I usually tell someone right away.
2. **W**   I keep a journal.
3. **MW** I often take notes, although I do not always refer to them.
4. **W**   I take good notes, then rewrite them at a later time.
5. **R**   I read in my free time.
6. **L**   I have the TV on even if I am not watching it.
7. **S**   I have good intentions of writing to people but usually call instead.
8. **V**   I often shut my eyes to help myself concentrate.
9. **M**   When studying or solving a problem, I pace back and forth.
10. **L**   I would rather hear a book on audiocassette than read it myself.
11. **V**   Forget the cassette, I would rather wait until it comes out on film.
12. **R**   I prefer reading the newspaper to watching the news on TV.
13. **L**   I prefer to study in a quiet setting.
14. **V**   To remember a spelling, I "see" the word in my mind.
15. **S**   I would prefer an oral exam to a written one.
16. **V**   I prefer a multiple choice format on a test.
17. **M**   I would rather do a project than write a paper.
18. **S**   I would rather give an oral report than a written one.

19. **R**   I remember better what I read rather than what I hear.
20. **W**   I keep a personal organizer.
21. **R**   I reread my notes several times.
22. **W**   I would rather take notes from the text than attend a lecture on the material.
23. **SL** I often "talk to myself."
24. **SL** I learn best when I study with a partner.
25. **V**   I can locate a passage that I have read by "seeing it."
26. **M**   I find it hard to sit still when I study.
27. **M**   If I forgot why I walked into the kitchen, I retrace my steps from the bedroom.
28. **V**   Once in bed for the night, I shut my eyes and plan the next day.
29. **L**   I cannot clean unless the music is on.
30. **R**   I would rather read directions than have someone tell me about them.
31. **R**   I can put something together as long as the directions are written.

Tally the number of S, W, M, R, L, and V responses and record the total in the following table.

S	W	M	R	L	V

If you have three or more responses of one letter, you most likely have a strong preference for that learning style. Most people have at least one strength, but you may have more than one.

RESULTS

Speaking (S): Three or more checks in this area indicate a preference for learning information by saying it. You may wish to read your notes and text aloud, or at least the chapter headings. It may be beneficial for you to have a study partner, or to speak into a tape recorder and play your tape back. You may ask someone to listen to you as you explain a principle. After reviewing information, play the part of a teacher by asking questions aloud. Repeat concepts aloud and ask questions of others.

Writing (W): Take notes from readings. Rewrite your notes on paper or index cards. Make tests for yourself and take them. Write notes in the margins of your text and notebooks.

Manipulative (M): Often thought of as the kinesthetic modality, learning occurs best by "doing." If you have this type of preference, make a model, map, or diagram of the information you need to learn. Write information on a black/white board. Carry index cards with the information you are trying to learn with you, and pull out the cards while you are walking, exercising, or cooking dinner. Draw answers in the air as you try to memorize information. Move your lips while reading or thinking.

Reading (R): Read and reread information if this is your preferred learning style. Ask to borrow other students' notes so you can read them and fill in any information you may have missed. Highlight text passages to easily locate information. Read chapter titles, headings, and summaries.

Listening (L): You would benefit from having a study group or at least a partner. To the extent possible, have others read to you. Tape lectures and review sessions whenever possible. Make review tapes for yourself and listen to them. Read and repeat information aloud after you have read or heard it. Call classmates and have them read their notes to you or quiz you over the phone.

Visualizing (V): If this is your learning strength, you learn best by picturing information in your head. You are apt to "see" a page of information. It is to your benefit to study, shut your eyes, and then recall the information. Take note of the way the information is written, as well as the shape, color, and size of the paper. This will help you recall the information later. Also picture yourself taking the exam, walking in, and calmly sitting down. This will help steady your nerves.

Often it is beneficial for you to study in more than one way. Remember, your learning profile is unique and just because your friend studies best when listening to music does not mean that the same will apply to you. Take a moment to inventory your strengths and develop a plan based on the way you learn best.

GETTING ORGANIZED TO STUDY

How much time do you have to study, or how much time are you willing to give based on your work schedule, information remembered from classes, anxiety level, and other commitments? Fill out the following time log to visually see how you have been spending your time. If possible, do this for several days, including Saturday and Sunday.

TIME LOG			
Day			
6:00 to 7:00 a.m.			
7:00 to 8:00			
8:00 to 9:00			
9:00 to 10:00			
10:00 to 11:00			
11:00 to 12:00 noon			
12:00 to 1:00 p.m.			
1:00 to 2:00			
2:00 to 3:00			
3:00 to 4:00			
4:00 to 5:00			
5:00 to 6:00			
6:00 to 7:00			
7:00 to 8:00			
8:00 to 9:00			
9:00 to 10:00			
10:00 to 11:00			

Based on how your time is usually spent, what available time do you have for studying? Will you be better off studying for a block of time in the afternoon or for several chunks throughout the day? Perhaps your schedule is such that you can only study on weekends. How much time can you commit to studying during your free time? Based on the amount of time you have, make a plan of when you are going to study. (You can always modify it later.)

STUDY TIME COMMITMENTS

Next, make a list of the supplies you will need for studying. This may sound nerdy, but it is a lot more fun studying if you have colored index cards and a candy supply.

STUDY SUPPLIES

Suggested Study Supplies	Your List of Study Supplies
Reference books (DSM-IV, texts, guides, dictionary, etc.)	
Assorted colored index cards	
Index cards on a wire	
Notetabs	
Assorted colored highlighters	
Timer/clock	
Goal sheet: long- and short-term	
Writing instruments	
Tissues	
Water or beverage	
Tape recorder	
Lined/unlined paper	
Snacks or treats	
Tools of the trade (goniometer, etc.)	
Class notes and prior exams if available	
Rabbit's foot or other good luck charms	

Stock your study area with the supplies you determined were needed. If you travel to the library or study in several different places, prepare a bag with your supplies so you will always have them on hand. Note: If you have run out of snacks more than three times, you need to re-evaluate your priorities!

Now that you have determined when you will study and what you need to begin, you are ready to make a plan of attack. Begin by developing a goal sheet for yourself. Examine the sample as a guideline for your goal sheet.

SAMPLE GOAL SHEET

Outcome Goal: *To pass NBCOT exam and become an OT*

Current Date	Objectives	Target Completion Date	Revision of Goals or Progress Notes
11/30	Complete 30 questions from review manual	11/30	Done. Got 23 correct.
12/1	Photocopy Amy's notes on TBI; give her copy of my SCI notes	12/2	
12/4	Read chapter summaries in textbook	12/4	Took longer than expected. Finished 12/5.
12/6	Make flashcards/vocab cards	12/6	Ran out of cards. Go shopping by 12/8.
12/9	Tape record content outline from text	12/11	Done. Victorious!
12/10	Finish vocab cards	12/10	Done. Pat self on back.
12/12	Highlight vocab in text	12/15	Finished 12/13. See a movie.
12/15	Reorganize notebook	12/16	No interest. Try again.
12/16	Form a study group	12/18	No problem.
12/17	Reorganize notebook	12/18	Watched TV instead.
12/19	Reorganize notebook	12/19	Maybe tomorrow.

Now complete your goal sheet.

GOAL SHEET			
Outcome Goal:			
Current Date	Objectives	Target Completion Date	Revision of Goals or Progress Notes

Review and revise your plan of attack often. If nothing else, remove the sheet from the book and post it where it will remind you that you do have a goal in mind. Be flexible. Your great aunt may stop over (and you know what that means) or you may find yourself completing goals ahead of schedule.

Make goals reasonable. It is unrealistic to expect yourself to complete 300 review questions in an hour, yet completing five vocabulary flashcards per week is no great accomplishment. Base your goals on the amount of overall time you have (and are willing) to study. Chapter One has a countdown calendar to help set your goals.

SPECIFIC STUDY AND TEST SKILLS

Reading comprehension: Points on the exam are not awarded for how long you study, your effort, or the amount of pages you read. Generally, grades are earned by knowing the correct information. It is quite important then that you have good comprehension of the material you are reading. Following are suggestions to aid in understanding your reading material.

1. Preview the chapter you are about to read by scanning the title, headings, introduction, summary, and, on occasion, the topic sentence in each paragraph. This can also be helpful to review a chapter or passage you have already read.
2. Take regular breaks to mentally review what you have read.
3. Turn topic sentences into questions.
4. Answer these in your head or jot them down for later review.
5. Read the material carefully, checking your understanding as you go along.

Note taking: Taking notes on material that you are studying can be beneficial. Remember, even if you never review the notes you take, the process of jotting them down can be helpful. Outlining with highlighters may help zero in on the main idea. If this method works well for you, use a different colored marker to highlight the details or supporting ideas. Reread your highlighted passages. Class notes can be highlighted as well as textbooks. Use margin notes to organize what you have read. Pay attention to key words or write questions in the margin for later review. Margin notes will help avoid wasted time searching for an answer because the explanation will be right there. Another way to take notes on important material is to jot down information in a separate notebook. Again, this is particularly helpful for those who learn best kinesthetically. Note taking should always be done by using phrases rather than complete sentences. Make an informal outline by writing down the main idea from a passage and several supporting details under the idea. Always jot down the page number or source of information so you can refer back to it if needed.

If you have found that you remember information best by picturing the words on a page or by writing, then you might consider mapping as a note-taking strategy. Draw a circle in the middle of your page and write the main idea in it. Write the major points regarding your main topic on connecting lines. This might include information such as causes and effects or symptoms and treatments. Add lines to your major points to connect minor details. See Figure 2-1 for an occupational therapy mapping example.

Lastly, notes can be written on index cards. Put one key concept on each notecard with supporting details. Reference your card so you know where to find additional information should you have a question. Write down vocabulary pertinent to the concept on your card. If there is a definition associated with your concept, write that on the back of your card so you can test yourself. One advantage to using notecards is the opportunity to put a few in your pocket to review when you are waiting for your ride, to stick on your mirror while you dry your hair, or to view on the refrigerator as you contemplate a snack.

Memory strategies: Comprehending the material you hear and read is one thing, but memorizing it is another. Fortunately, most of what is asked of us deals more with integrating and applying information rather than memorizing long lists of terms. However, there are occasions when you will be responsible for producing an exact definition, listing the components of a subject, or remembering several general concepts. If you can recite the alphabet, then you should be able to remember just about anything. Consider all the similar sounding letters in the alphabet (B, C, D, E, G, P, T, V, Z), yet even with confusing sounds we have mastered the ABCs. Most likely, you were able to learn the alphabet because of repetition. Chances are you know a little tune whereby you can sing the ABCs on demand. The same strategies, plus some others, that worked when you were 5 years old can work for you now.

We are constantly taking in information, but the degree to which we remember or retrieve the information depends on several factors. Exposure or repetition is definitely a factor that affects our ability to remember an item. For instance, fill in the following:

"Meet George Jetson, his boy _____."
"That's the way we all became the _____ Bunch."
"It takes one to _____ one."
"I've been_____ on the railroad."

You have heard these phrases over and over until you automatically know the answer. Overlearning is an effective way to move information from your short-term memory to your long-term knowledge. Read and reread the information you are trying to memorize. Once you feel you have learned the material, review it regularly to refresh your memory. Each time you review the material, it will take less and less time until you can anticipate words and phrases before you even read them. As you review material, recite it so you can see and hear the information. Writing and rewriting (more than once) will help you to retain information. Try to link new information with prior knowledge.

Use rhymes, acronyms, acrostics, and substitutions in familiar sayings or tunes. For instance, if you are trying to memorize the joints in the hands (MCP, PIP, DIP), you might memorize My Cousin Paul Put Ice Pieces Down Ida's Pants. Rearrange items in your list (unless they have to be remembered in a specific order) to make it easier to work with.

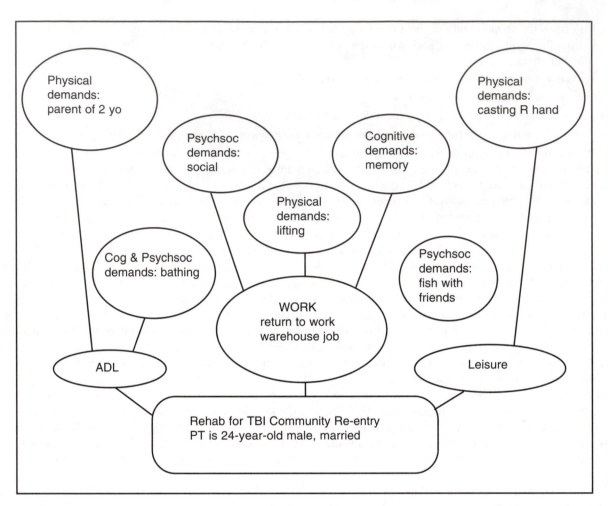

Figure 2-1. Occupational therapy mapping example.

Test-taking strategies: Know the format of the test. It is easier to prepare when you know what the expectations are. For instance, on an essay test, you will have to retrieve information and do so in an orderly way. You will need to know pertinent vocabulary and how to use it appropriately. However, the reason you are reading this book is because of a certain little multiple choice test that is coming to a testing center near you. A multiple choice format is advantageous in that you need only to recognize the correct answer rather than generate it yourself. Still, there are techniques that will enhance your chances of choosing the correct answer. The following are some tactics that will:

    A. Help you to buy a new car

    B. Help you lose 10 pounds

    C. Get you a date with you-know-who

    D. Help you succeed on the big test

The correct answer is D, the following test-taking strategies will help you succeed on the exam.

- Plan your time: Divide your time by the number of questions. Leave several minutes' leeway.

- Read the entire question: Anticipate the answer but do not be impulsive. Read each answer thoroughly before choosing.

- Respond to each question: If you leave it blank, it is definitely wrong. If you have absolutely no clue, then make the best guess possible. Check to make sure you keyed it correctly.

- If you are unsure of the answer: Narrow it down by eliminating the responses you know are incorrect. Sometimes you can get clues from reading other questions.

- Pay particular attention to qualifying words: Words such as *except, most, best, least,* and *not.*

- Do not overinterpret the questions: Read them at face value.

- If you do not know the right answer: Make the best response possible and put a check by the question. If you have the time, return to the question to recheck. Do not waste time on the questions you do not know.
- If you must skip a question: Flag it. Again, you are better off answering all questions and flagging the ones you want to check later.
- Trust your instincts: Do not second guess yourself. Be cautious about changing answers.
- Check the time: Check the clock or your watch occasionally to make sure you are on target.

READY TO STUDY

With supplies at hand, snacks in stock, and goal sheet pinned to your chest, you are ready to get down and dirty. Before you sit down, you need to decide on a place for your intellectual experience (study environment). Consider the amount of noise, light, temperature, and physical comfort of your study area. In addition, will there be visual interference that will cause you to look up every few moments? Is your studying most effective morning, noon, or night? Make these decisions now to maximize your effectiveness. Refer to your goal list to set expectations for each particular study session. Be aware that the first few minutes of your session are considered warm-up time that you will spend "shifting gears" and getting in the right mindset. Monitor your progress to check for fatigue and mind wandering. Evaluate your session afterward to see if you were effective or if you need to change something for next time. Refer to the following study session evaluation checklist:

1. Did I have specific goals in mind as I sat down to study?
2. Were my expectations realistic?
3. Did I accomplish what I set out to do?
4. Was the time I set aside enough?
5. Did I implement specific study techniques based on my preferred learning style?
6. Was I distracted or tired?

TROUBLE-SHOOTING

If your efforts are sincere but you are not getting the results you desire, refer to the following problem-solving solutions.

TROUBLE-SHOOTING SOLUTIONS	
If:	Try:
You are sleepy	Physical activity, a break, a real nap, fresh air, a study partner, speaking aloud.
Your mind wanders	A new location; earplugs; set smaller, more obtainable goals; use manipulatives.
You are bored	Vary your routine, give yourself rewards, try 15 minutes on/15 minutes off, switch from reading to writing to speaking.
There are too many interruptions	Take the phone off the hook/turn the answering machine on, put up a sign that says "Great mind at work—Please do not interrupt."
You are worried, overwhelmed	Break down tasks to even smaller chunks, see Relaxation Techniques.
You are forgetting previously learned material	Use clues to get information flowing, review less material more frequently, do not move to new concepts until old concepts are mastered, try learning through a different modality.
You are behind on your goals	Re-evaluate your time, double up on goals, refer to Chapter One for countdown calendar.

RELAXATION TECHNIQUES AND COPING SKILLS

As an occupational therapy student you have learned that relaxation techniques are effective for helping your patients to cope. Studying for the exam is a good time to use relaxation exercises yourself. The following exercises may be effective both before and during the exam.

Self talk: Ask yourself what is the worst thing that will happen if you do not study tonight or if you do not pass the test. Tell yourself that you can do this. You have done other difficult things and can do this, too. You are great!

Review successes: Remind yourself of previous successes. You have made it this far. You have passed all your courses. You have passed other exams. You have completed a successful affiliation.

Take inventory: Do you know more than you did last year? Do you know more than you did last month? Have you studied/reviewed material recently?

Develop support systems: Let people know of your goals. Phone others to discuss your concerns. Be with people who will validate your self-worth.

Visualization: Picture yourself walking into the exam with confidence. Visualize yourself getting the results in the mail and scoring in the top 20%.

Daydream: Think about tanning on the beach or skiing down a slope. Take a vacation in your mind.

Physical activity: Walking can clear your head and relax your muscles. Elevate your feet by lying on the floor and placing your feet on a chair for 10 minutes.

Deep breathing: Try deep cleansing breaths. Shut your eyes and slowly inhale through your nose. Hold the breath for 3 to 5 seconds, then exhale through your mouth. Repeat every time you feel stressed. If you are familiar with meditation techniques, try that after a few deep cleansing breaths.

SUMMARY

There is a satisfaction in knowing that one has done his or her best. The ideas presented in this chapter are suggestions to help you reach your goal of preparing, studying, and ultimately passing your examination. Preparing to study according to your strengths and weaknesses is an important part of studying effectively. Information regarding learning styles, organization, and specific study strategies is included in this chapter. It is important to develop the strategies that will be of most benefit to you. A study plan will ultimately help you save time and learn efficiently and effectively.

Chapter Three

Study Content Outlines

In this chapter you will find three outlines that cover content topics on the exam. Each study outline covers content in one of three areas: physical management, mental health/cognitive management, and administration management. Special attention must be paid to the interaction of the physical and mental health management outlines. Expert occupational therapists know that pathology is not just physical or psychiatric. In addition, many other areas overlap, such as occupational performance, frame of reference, impact of illness on function, and normal development. Be sure to review all the outlines for a more complete overview. Other ways to make your own context outline include your class notes, tables of contents from textbooks, and resources such as Sladyk's *OT Study Cards in a Box* or Reed's *Quick Reference to Occupational Therapy.*

As a student studying for the exam, you may want to use these outlines to develop your study plan or to double check your content after studying. It is natural to miss "depth" in areas you are weak, so use the outline to make sure your study plan is whole.

PHYSICAL MANAGEMENT CONTENT OUTLINE

I.   Systems Review
    A. Structure and function of circulatory, respiratory, digestive, excretory, nervous

II. Tissue Types
    A. Connective tissue
        1. Tendons, ligaments, bone, cartilage

III. Joint Classification
    A. Diarthrodial/synovial
        1. Uniaxial, biaxial, triaxial
    B. Synarthrodial
    C. Amphiarthrodial

IV. Tissue Reaction to Disease and Injury
    A. Inflammation/edema
        1. Redness, pain, swelling, heat, decreased function
    B. Repair, healing stages

V.   Causes of Disease, Disorders, and Function
    A. Etiology classifications
        1. Hereditary, congenital, traumatic, physical
        2. Chemical, infectious, inflammation, vascular, metabolic
        3. Nutritional, psychological, iatrogenic, idiopathic, tumors

VI. Frames of Reference

    A. Biomechanical

        1. Evaluation assesses physical limitations, ROM, strength, endurance

        2. Treatment to restore function

    B. Occupational performance

        1. Evaluation of performance components including sensorimotor, neuromuscular, motor, cognitive, psycho-social

        2. Treatment areas include activities of daily living, work, play/leisure

            a. Stage one: remediate performance components

            b. Stage two: enabling activities

            c. Stage three: purposeful activity

            d. Stage four: community reintegration

    C. Rehabilitation and Neurodevelopmental approaches

        1. Evaluation of abilities

        2. Treatment is restorative, acquisition of role performance

        3. Sensorimotor

        4. Evaluation of central nervous system dysfunction

        5. Treatment focus is sensory input, which leads to motor output, Rood, Bobath, Brunnstrom, PNF

        6. Motor learning

VII. General Concerns of All Disorders

    A. Effects of inactivity on neuromuscular, musculoskeletal, digestive, respiratory, skin, cardiovascular, renal, psychosocial

VIII. Amputations

    A. Health concerns: etiology can be peripheral vascular disease, diabetes, trauma, COPD, cardiac problems

    B. OT concerns: preprosthetic training, healing issues, cosmesis versus cosmetic, phantom pain, body image, prosthetic training, skin and stump care, donning and doffing, scar massage, adaptation, self-care, work, leisure, sexual adjustment

IX. Arthritis and Other Connective Tissue Diseases

    A. Health concerns: disease process, systemic versus nonsystemic, inflammatory versus noninflammatory, rapid versus insidious, exacerbation and remissions, secondary complications

    B. OT concerns: mobility and function, deformity, contractures, joint protection and body mechanics, adaptive equipment, energy conservation, work simplification, support group referral, rest, adapt home and work site, psychological support, sexual adjustment, family education

X. Burns

    A. Health concerns: classification; rule of nines; percent of total body surface area; first-degree superficial; second-degree partial thickness; third-degree full thickness; fourth-degree electrical; débridement; auto; full or split thickness grafts; shock; complications including pulmonary, metabolic, cardiac

    B. OT concerns: acute phase includes aseptic techniques, infection control, débridement; rehabilitation phase includes hypertrophic scarring, heterotrophic bone ossification, pressure gradient therapy; position of comfort may cause deformity; splints for oral, neck, elbow, axilla, hand, ankle; psychosocial adjustment; self-image; locus of control; community reentry

XI. Cancer

A. Health concerns: improved diagnostic techniques including CT scan, PET scan, MRI; prognosis varies by age, neurological status, tumor size, stage or grade, metastatic tumor from another site; treatments include surgery, radiation, chemotherapy

B. OT concerns: restorative, supportive, palliative intervention; self-care; fatigue; ostomy care; mobility; pain; fear of recurrence; community involvement; vocational issues; hospice care; family education; home modification

XII. Cardiac Dysfunction

A. Health concerns: medical history, shortness of breath, angina, metabolic equivalent (MET) levels, dyspnea, blood pressure, very light activity to 100 heart rate, avoid valsalva's maneuver, arrhythmia

B. OT concerns: lifestyle, avocational interests, stress, adjustment to limitations, energy conservation, work simplification, graded exercise routine, psychosocial adjustment, family education, safety, role adjustments

XIII. Cerebral Palsy

A. Health concerns: prenatal, perinatal, postnatal; tone is mixed, spastic, or dystonic; athetoid; ataxia; praxis, oral motor, feeding problems; dysarthria; mental retardation possible

B. OT concerns: sensory processing, developmental delays, primitive reflex activity, bilateral integration, ADLs, early intervention, school intervention and inclusion, play, family support and education, wheelchair positioning, splinting, adaptive equipment, home modifications

XIV. Cerebral Vascular Accident

A. Health concerns: thrombus, embolus, aneurysm, hemorrhage, transient ischemic attack (TIA), anoxia, middle cerebral artery, lesion side has contralateral hemiplegia, reflex sympathetic dystrophy

B. OT concerns: left CVA may include right hemiplegia or hemiparesis; apraxia; hemianopsia; impaired sequencing skills; be slow or cautious; show receptive, expressive, or global aphasia. Right CVA may include left hemiplegia or hemiparesis; hemianopsia; visual spatial deficits; left in attention; position in space problems; denial of illness. All CVAs may show sensory loss; synergy; tone; decreased function in ADLs, work, leisure. Changed self-image, isolation, home modification, driver training, adaptive equipment, safety, family education

XV. Chronic Pain Conditions

A. Health concerns: noscioceptive or persistent pain, abusing pain medication

B. OT concerns: maladaptive responses, depression, withdrawal from roles, conditioning exercises, work hardening, stress reduction, leisure activities, supportive environment, positive self-talk, visualization, self-hypnosis, imagery, nutrition, family support

XVI. Guillain-Barré and Motor Unit Diseases

A. Health concerns: demyelination, spinal nerve roots, peripheral nerves

B. OT concerns: sensory loss, muscle atrophy, contractures, fatigue, endurance, oral motor function, respiratory problems, decreased trunk control, fine and gross motor coordination, ataxia, pain, psychosocial adjustments, home modifications, ADLs, work and leisure, incomplete recovery

XVII. Hand Injuries

A. Health concerns: joint injuries and deformities; tendon injuries; nerve compression and injuries in median, radial, or ulnar nerves; muscle imbalance; atrophy or weakness

B. OT concerns: loss of sensation; decreased functional grasp and pinch; sensory discrimination; fine motor skills; loss of function in ADLs, work, leisure; correct splint for specific diagnoses

XVIII. Head Injuries

A. Health concerns: orthopedic such as fractures, heterotopic ossification, neurological, coupe and countercoupe, cerebral contusions, frontal and temporal lobe involvement common, cranial nerves, coma and altered level of consciousness, amnesia, seizures, hydrocephalus

B. OT concerns: sensory loss; visual perceptual and vision changes; cognitive executive function; motoric loss; behavioral changes; aphasia; dysphagia; self-care; work productivity; leisure; adaptive equipment; splints; driver training; family education; safety in motor, cognitive, behavior

XIX. Hip Fracture

A. Health concerns: total hip arthroplasty, arthrodesis, total hip articular replacement with internal eccentric shells, restricted mobility, pain, age as an issue

B. OT concerns: mobility, independence, fear of reinjury, adaptive equipment, loss of roles, home modification, endurance, adaptive equipment

XX. Multiple Sclerosis and Other Degenerative Diseases

A. Health concerns: CNS disorder, exacerbation and remission, unpredictable process

B. OT concerns: muscle weakness, incoordination, tremors, sensory loss, pain, proprioception loss, visual disturbances including diplopia, dysarthria, bladder problems, psychological adjustment including depression and euphoria, cognitive involvement, support group referral, home and work site adaptations, safety issues, adaptive equipment, family education, ongoing driving evaluation

XXI. Muscular Dystrophy

A. Health concerns: genetic disorder, major progressive muscle weakness, atrophy of limbs and trunk, pulmonary problems, Gowers' sign, lordosis, scoliosis, fat replaces muscle, cardiac complications, scapula winging

B. OT concerns: prevent contractures, splinting, adaptive equipment, muscle imbalance, ADLs, school intervention and inclusion, play, gait disturbances, mild cognitive problems, maintain function, family support and education, wheelchair positioning, home modifications

XXII. Spinal Cord Injuries

A. Health concerns: orthopedic, neurological, cardiopulmonary, autonomic dysreflexia, postural hypotension, decreased temperature regulation

B. OT concerns: sensory loss, splints, body image, bowel and bladder function, strengthening, personal relationships, sexual readjustment, self-care, work productivity, leisure, home modification, adaptive equipment, driver education, family education

XXIII. Spina Bifida

A. Health concerns: failure of fusion, neural arches, meningocele, open or closed sac, surgery, infection, hydrocephalus

B. OT concerns: gross motor and developmental disturbances, self-care, school intervention and inclusion, adaptive equipment, wheelchair positioning, home modifications, family support and education

MENTAL HEALTH/COGNITIVE MANAGEMENT CONTENT OUTLINE

I. Normal Development

  A. Life cycle theory

    1. Piaget, Gesell, Sullivan, Kohlberg, Freud, Erikson

    2. Stages, landmarks, crisis points, cultural impact

  B. Developmental theory

    1. Physical, cognitive, emotional milestones from birth to death

II. Frames of Reference

A. Behavioral

1. Evaluation is of adaptive or maladaptive behaviors

2. Treatment based on classical and operant conditioning. Techniques such as shaping, chaining, token economy, biofeedback are used to reinforce desired behavior

B. Cognitive behavioral

1. Evaluation of self-regulation and self-control

2. Treatment involves reinforcement, modeling, observation; develop insight and understanding; modify how person thinks

C. Cognitive disability

1. Evaluation is on assessing cognitive functioning level

2. Treatment is based on brain pathology, match activities to cognitive level by changing activity not person, function exists when person is capable of meeting routine task demands

D. Developmental

1. Evaluation is of specific stages that are progressive and hierarchical

2. Treatment addresses developmental themes, groups are based on different levels, drive toward mastery, skills must be learned in sequence of normal development

E. Model of human occupation

1. Evaluation looks at volition, habituation, performance

2. Treatment based on the human as an open system that can change through interaction with the environment, competency is based on ability to perform daily tasks, directive groups

F. Psychodynamic

1. Evaluation of unconscious conflict; aspects of personality, id, ego, superego

2. Treatment integrates wants, needs, drives in conscious awareness; object relations; transference and counter transference; defenses; therapeutic sense of self

G. Sensory integration

1. Evaluation is of brain's ability to filter, organize, integrate sensory information; look for mature adaptive responses

2. Treatment is based on neuroscience, neuropsychology, neurophysiology; vestibular, tactile, proprioceptive input impacts postural control, body schema, bonding, coordination, language, perception, emotions and is base for visual and auditory functions, related to learning disabilities in children, process is developmental

H. Occupation-based theories

1. Evaluation of person, environment, occupations

2. Treatment is person centered addressing roles and activities client has as goals, adapt environment to meet needs

I. Therapeutic process

1. Patient/therapist relationship

a. Counseling skills, ethics, confidentiality

2. Environment

a. Structured versus unstructured, hospital, community milieu, group homes

3. Role of occupational therapy on a multidisciplinary team

a. Role of other members on treatment team

III. Alcohol and Other Substance Abuse

A. Health concerns: difference between abuse and dependency; effects on CNS; etiology includes genetic, neurochemical, environmental factors; slippage is common

B. OT concerns: assess suicidal potential; vocational, social, leisure components mostly impacted; dual diagnosis with another mental health disability; transference and counter transference are often magnified

IV. Alzheimer's and Other Dementia Disorders

A. Health concerns: etiology includes neurochemical, environmental, viral, trauma, genetic, substance abuse

B. OT concerns: awareness, orientation, organization, attention, problem solving, decision making, reasoning, insight, judgment, functional adaptation, supervision needed, remedial techniques, safety, perceptual problems may not be apparent at first, family education and support

V. Anxiety Disorders

A. Health concerns: anxiety can be mild to severe, anti-anxiety medication helpful, post-traumatic stress disorder (PTSD) always stems from a trauma

B. OT concerns: assess suicidal potential; avoidance behaviors shown; occupational and social functioning impaired; behavioral techniques such as relaxation, desensitization, imagery effective

VI. Attention Deficit Disorder (ADD) and Attention Deficit Hyperactivity Disorder (ADHD)

A. Health concerns: etiology may be neurological in combination with environmental factors, medication

B. OT concerns: low stimulation environment, mastery of developmental skills, self-regulation, self-advocacy skills, family education, inclusion in school

VII. Bipolar Disorder, Depression, and Other Affective Disorders

A. Health concerns: familial patterns are common, depression is most common of all psychiatric disorders, medications such as an anti-depressant and lithium manage symptoms

B. OT concerns: assess suicidal potential, use precautions due to decreased judgment, may affect all performance areas especially social, activities need to be gratifying

VIII. Eating Disorders

A. Health concerns: include anorexia nervosa and bulimia, medical management of weight, etiology usually includes family dysfunction, nutritional needs, biological changes, may be chronic and lifetime disease

B. OT concerns: assess suicidal potential; personality traits include decreased self-esteem, perfectionism, need for control; food is major focus, develop interest in activities; social skills and leisure are critical areas

IX. Mental Retardation/Pervasive Developmental Disorder (PDD)

A. Health concerns: Down syndrome or other genetic causes, other disabilities such as seizures or physical issues, medications

B. OT concerns: sensory and neurodevelopmental approaches to minimize physical problems and encourage developmental skills, social skills training, vocational training, family support, inclusion, ADL and leisure education, sexual education

X. Learning Issues

A. Health concerns: etiology may be neurological or orthopedic, school performance

B. OT concerns: appropriate learning, mastery of developmental skills, self-advocacy skills, family education, accommodations and inclusion in the classroom

XI. Personality Disorders

A. Health concerns: lifelong patterns, inaccurate perception of self and others

B. OT concerns: assess suicidal potential; poor personal values and goals; relationship problems; individual versus group treatment depends on disorder; transference and counter transference; vocational, social, leisure are mostly affected

XII. Schizophrenia and Other Psychotic Disorders

A. Health concerns: thought disorder including hallucinations and delusions, positive versus negative symptoms, often chronic in nature, medication side effects such as tardive dyskinesia and extrapyramidal symptoms

B. OT concerns: assess suicidal potential, all performance areas are affected, do not challenge psychotic thinking, address sensorimotor and cognitive disabilities, behavioral techniques, medication regime

XIII. Occupational Therapy Groups

A. Theory

1. Fidler's task-oriented, Mosey and Llorens' developmental, Allen's cognitive levels, Kaplan's directive, Ross' structured five stage, Howe and Schwartzberg's functional groups

B. Group or individual treatment topic examples by performance components

1. Sensorimotor

a. Sensory integration and movement groups

2. Cognitive

a. Task and project groups

3. Psychosocial

a. Creative and projective arts groups

C. Group or individual treatment topic examples by performance areas

1. ADLs

a. Social skills, sexual expression, grooming, time management, dressing, cooking

2. Work and productive activities

a. Prevocational, work exploration, work hardening, parenting, retirement, home making, sensory integration, play, coping skills, assertiveness

3. Play or leisure

a. Play, dance, music, arts and crafts, leisure exploration, recreation

ADMINISTRATION MANAGEMENT CONTENT OUTLINE

I. Program Development

A. Models of practice; medical-, community-, school-based

B. Needs assessment

1. Focus group, demographics, key informants, survey, questionnaire, using research

C. Program planning

1. Philosophy, mission statement, goals, objectives

D. Treatment

1. Referral, screening, assessment, intervention plan, intervention including direct and consulting, transition services, discontinuation

E. Program evaluation

II. Program Management

A. Management by objectives (MBO); organizational policies including ADA and OBRA; accreditation requirements including JCAHO, CARE, state requirements

B. Documentation

1. Objective versus subjective, identify patient's strengths and weaknesses

2. Requirements; format including SOAP, POMR, narrative

C. Reimbursement

1. DRGs, Medicare Part A, Medicare Part B; Tri-Alliance; private third-party payers, including nonprofit and for profit; HMOs; worker's compensation

D. Quality assurance and continuous quality improvement

E. Budget and financial aspects

    1. Supplies and equipment, direct versus indirect, capital expenses, fixed versus variable expenses

F. OT promotion and marketing

G. Ethics

    1. Reporting violations

H. Standards of practice

I. Safety standards

    1. Universal precautions, environmental health, incident reports

J. Continuing education

    1. Update theories and techniques

K. Patient rights

    1. Confidentiality, refuse treatment

L. Research

    1. Benefits and use in daily practice, evidence-based practice

M. AOTA, AOTF, NBCOT

III. Personnel Management

A. OT personnel and credentialing OT, OTA, OT aide

B. Productivity

    1. Measurement methods and performance appraisals

C. Supervision

D. Staff retention

E. Functions of an OT

    1. Role delineation of OT and OTA

    2. Collaboration of the OT and OTA

F. Malpractice and liability

IV. Community versus Medical Models

V. Wellness and Health Promotion

A. Lifestyle redesign

B. Emerging practice

Chapter Four

Fieldwork Experience as a Study Guide

ROLE OF FIELDWORK

The purpose of fieldwork is to integrate classroom study with clinical practice and develop clinical reasoning skills. To help you use your fieldwork experience to study for the exam, you must first understand some of the policies established by AOTA.

Fieldwork in an accredited OT school is divided into two types: Level I and Level II. Level I fieldwork is experienced during your studies, usually done part-time during the academic year. Level II is typically full-time, after you have completed your studies. Of course, due to the shortages of fieldwork sites, your school may have provided you with a creative, nontraditional Level II fieldwork. Although these fieldwork experiences are different from what has been traditional in the past, it is our experience that these students do equally well on the exam.

Much of what you know as an occupational therapy student was developed and refined during your fieldwork experiences. This section of the book is designed to help you review your fieldwork experience. We have provided opportunities to reflect on your areas of accomplishment and those that need further review before you take the exam. Begin by identifying all of your fieldwork sites using the example below.

SAMPLE FIELDWORK REVIEW			
Fieldwork Sites	*Level I*	*Level II*	*On My Own*
St. Mary's Hospital	Observed hand tx		Observed peds
Community Mental Health Center		Community skills assessments	
Summer Program for Special Kids			Helped OT run SI groups

Use the following table to identify your fieldwork experiences. Fill in each square with a brief summary of what you did at each fieldwork site. Include Levels I and II fieldwork and any additional experiences you have had working with an OT.

FIELDWORK REVIEW			
Fieldwork Sites	*Level I*	*Level II*	*On My Own*

Now that you have reviewed your fieldwork experiences, it is time to look at the variety of consumers with which you have worked. Below is a table of diagnostic categories with which many OTs work. It is not expected that you have had experiences in all these areas. On the contrary, students who focused their experiences in limited areas developed clinical reasoning more easily. This table is designed to point out in which areas you are accomplished and which areas you may need to review before the exam. Use a check mark to indicate your assessment of your fieldwork experience. Blank spaces are provided at the end of the table to add other diagnostic categories.

FIELDWORK DIAGNOSIS REVIEW					
Diagnosis	No Experience	Observation Experience	Some Experience	A Lot of Experience	Community vs. Inpatient Model
AIDS/infectious diseases					
Amputation					
Arthritis					
Bipolar disorder					
Burns					
Cancer					
Cardiac disease					
Cerebral palsy					
Child/elder abuse					
CVA/neurological issues					
Dementia					
Depression					
Diabetes					
Drug/alcohol abuse					
Eating disorders					
Failure to thrive					
Hand/arm conditions/splints					
Head injuries					
Kidney disease					
Learning issues/ADHD					
Mental retardation/PDD					
Multiple sclerosis					
Muscular dystrophy					
Orthopedic conditions					
Parkinson's disease					
Personality disorders					
Schizophrenia					
SI dysfunction					
Spina bifida					
Spinal cord injuries					
Visual issues					
Wellness					

After you have completed a review of your fieldwork experiences, it is time to make an assessment of the areas you need to review before the exam. Fieldwork was never intended to provide you with a view of all occupational therapy practice. It would be expected that many of your check marks on the fieldwork diagnosis review table would be in the "No Experience" column.

Setting studying priorities for the exam should begin in the "No Experience" and "Observation Experience" columns. Even with that as a starting place, you may feel like it is too much to manage at once. Use the study priorities chart to set your study priorities.

STUDY PRIORITIES			
Diagnosis	*Top Priority*	*Second Priority*	*No Need to Study*
AIDS/infectious diseases			
Amputation			
Arthritis			
Bipolar disorder			
Burns			
Cancer			
Cardiac disease			
Cerebral palsy			
Child/elder abuse			
CVA/neurological issues			
Dementia			
Depression			
Diabetes			
Drug/alcohol abuse			
Eating disorders			
Failure to thrive			
Hand/arm conditions/splints			
Head injuries			
Kidney disease			
Learning issues/ADHD			
Mental retardation/PDD			
Multiple sclerosis			
Muscular dystrophy			
Orthopedic conditions			
Parkinson's disease			
Personality disorders			
Schizophrenia			
SI dysfunction			
Spina bifida			
Spinal cord injuries			
Visual issues			
Wellness			

When reviewing the diagnoses you were exposed to during fieldwork also consider the modalities used. For example, you may have been exposed to hand injuries but have little experience with splinting because the facility had a non-OT specialist who did the splint construction for the clients. For each diagnosis, consider making your own study card that looks like this:

HAND INJURIES		
Diagnosis	*Treatments*	*Anatomy*
General issues	**Splinting issues:** Contour around bone Straps do not limit blood flow Custom splints for wounds Client education, wear schedule Consider cognitive and social issues **Edema issues:** Volumeter measurements Positioning Pain management **Functional roles:** Changes in roles including emotional issues	Preserve arches of hand Trauma and edema lead to deformity unless addressed Recovery time for nerves 1 inch per month **Peripheral nerve injury:** Muscle imbalance, deformity **Radial nerve injury:** Wrist drop, weak grasp **Median nerve injury:** Lateral three fingers affected, carpal tunnel syndrome **Ulnar nerve injury:** Impaired thumb, weak grasp
Carpel tunnel Arthritis Radial nerve palsy	Wrist cock up splint Functional assessment	Trim tip of thumb to allow movement
Crush trauma CVA SCI Burns Arthritis	Resting hand splint Functional assessment	Provides functional position Decreases tone in CVA Even padding to reduce pressure points
Median nerve injuries Thumb issues	Thumb spica splint Functional assessment	
Joint ROM or or soft tissue	Serial casting or dynamic splints	Force encourages movement Weak bones break with force

Now that you have set your topic priorities, consider the amount of time available before the exam and what time you have outside of your current responsibilities to study. Review Chapter Two and incorporate your priorities in your study plan. Next review Chapter 3, which outlines physical, mental health/cognitive, and administration management content.

When working on the study questions in the next section, you may find it helpful to recall some of your patients from your affiliations to problem solve the answer to a question. You can organize your study review notes based on classic symptoms versus clinical symptoms you saw on your affiliations. This will allow you to think through a question on the exam with a story visualization of what the patient would look like. Review the following example and then fill out your own table.

SAMPLE CLASSIC VERSUS CLINICAL PICTURES DURING FIELDWORK			
Diagnosis	Patient's First Name	Classic Symptoms	Clinical Symptoms Seen on Fieldwork
CVA-left cortex	Samuel	Expressive aphasia	Mild
		Receptive aphasia	Not present
		Right side weakness	Yes
		Spasticity	Yes, required splint
Schizophrenia	Anna	Withdrawn	No
		Flat affect	Blunted but not flat
		Hallucinations	Heard voices
		Delusions	No
		Poor hygiene	Good with reminder

Use the following table to outline your own patient stories. Fill in the spaces with the classic symptoms based on your class notes and textbooks. Picture the patient in your mind and fill in the clinical symptoms you saw during your fieldwork.

This exercise will help you answer exam questions using the clinical reasoning skills you developed during fieldwork. When faced with a question such as developing a treatment activity for a person with schizophrenia or a CVA, picture your patient trying each of the available answers. This might help you eliminate wrong answers and zero in on the correct answer.

SUMMARY

Reviewing your fieldwork experiences will help you recognize both accomplishments and areas that need further study. Examining each different diagnosis that you saw during both Level I and Level II fieldwork will help you to prioritize studying for the exam. Visualizing patient stories in your mind may help you eliminate wrong answers on the exam and remember correct ones.

CLASSIC VERSUS CLINICAL PICTURES DURING FIELDWORK			
Diagnosis	Patient's First Name	Classic Symptoms	Clinical Symptoms Seen on Fieldwork

SECTION III

Study Questions

Chapter Five

Mixed Domain, Task, and Knowledge Study Questions with Answers

GETTING DOWN TO BUSINESS

The NBCOT exam has a total of 200 questions and a time limit of 4 hours. This means that you need to answer 50 questions per hour. To help you get ready for the NBCOT exam, we have designed our study questions to simulate some of the factors you will notice when you take the real exam. First, we have divided our 600 study questions into 50-question sections. Although our study questions are different from the real exam questions, you can use them to pace yourself when studying. If you are working on pacing yourself, you should try to complete one section per hour. Consider using a timer or stopwatch. Second, we have mixed the topics of our study questions like the NBCOT exam. This means that you might answer a question on CVA followed by a question on group process. Answers and explanations for all the questions are available after each section.

Remember to read each study question carefully. Pay attention to detail words such as *except, most, best, least,* and *not*. The exam questions, as well as our study questions, are not trick questions. If you do not understand the question the first time you read it, read it again slowly. Do not overread a question.

STUDY QUESTIONS

Section One

1. The C-6 client you are working with complains of dizziness and nausea and seems to be losing consciousness as you bring him to standing in the standing table. Your *best* course of action is:

    A. Wait, the symptoms should pass as tolerance increases

    B. Bring him down to the wheelchair again

    C. Call for his nurse

    D. Bring him down to the wheelchair, then immediately recline him

2. A performance skill for a client in a low back pain program would be:

    A. Muscle strength

    B. Work tolerance

    C. Cognitive functioning

    D. Lifting tolerance

3. Choose the item that does *not* describe normal developmental expectations for an 8-year-old:
    A. Project level play is preferred
    B. Deductive reasoning is possible
    C. Playing dress up is a favored activity
    D. Has the ability to perceive and organize information

4. To be reimbursed under Medicare Part B, outpatient occupational therapy services must do all of the following *except*:
    A. Meet conditions set forth in coverage guidelines
    B. Services must be furnished under a written plan
    C. A physician must certify need for treatment
    D. The OT must be hospital affiliated

5. Inflammation of the common extensor origin of the forearm extensor musculature may result in:
    A. Gamekeeper's thumb
    B. Golfer's elbow
    C. Tennis elbow
    D. Pitcher's shoulder

6. An OT using the psychoanalytic frame of reference suggests kneading dough to make bread as an activity for a nonverbal and angry patient. The OT is basing her activity choice on which of the following concepts?
    A. Acting out
    B. Sublimation
    C. Identification
    D. Regression

7. *The Practice Framework* delineates and defines occupational therapy services. Which is *not* true of the framework?
    A. It provides a fee structure, flexible for use in different programs
    B. It is used by AOTA in many official documents
    C. It provides a base of consistent terminology
    D. It is updated periodically in accordance with current theory and practice

8. Entry-level OTAs are allowed to perform occupational therapy if supervised by:
    A. A nursing director
    B. A physician
    C. Another OTA who has experience
    D. An OT

9. Degenerative disorders commonly associated with depression, dementia, and psychosis include all of the following *except*:
    A. Parkinson's disease
    B. Huntington's disease
    C. Wilson's disease
    D. Connective tissue disease

10. Which ligament limits vertebral column extension?

    A. Posterior longitudinal ligament

    B. Ligamentum flavum

    C. Supraspinatus

    D. Anterior longitudinal ligament

11. In a 6-month-old child, symptoms such as abnormal muscle tone, delayed or exaggerated reflexes, postural abnormalities, and delayed motor development are signs of:

    A. Nothing to worry about, some 6-month-old children are like that

    B. Autism

    C. Mental retardation

    D. Cerebral palsy

12. Emotional flight in an emergency situation is dominated by which nervous system?

    A. Peripheral nervous system

    B. Sympathetic nervous system

    C. Parasympathetic nervous system

    D. Central nervous system

13. Direct occupational therapy services include:

    A. The OT as consultant

    B. A focus on wellness and prevention

    C. A hands-on, face-to-face relationship between the client and the therapist

    D. The OT as fieldwork supervisor

14. A patient who experiences abrupt changes and swings in emotional tone despite what is occurring in his or her external environment is *best* described as:

    A. Labile

    B. Anhedonic

    C. Inappropriate

    D. Euphoric

15. All of the following are clinical symptoms of spasticity *except*:

    A. A stretch reflex

    B. Clonus

    C. Atrophy

    D. Hyperactive tendon tap

16. A self-employed OT does contract work in several nursing homes. Who is responsible for malpractice and liability insurance?

    A. Each nursing home covers the OT while he or she is working at the facility

    B. AOTA covers the OT

    C. The state department of nursing home licensure covers the OT

    D. Each OT must carry individual coverage

17. Documentation of OT services to a patient should include all of the following *except*:
    A. The patient's response to treatment
    B. The treatment techniques used
    C. The patient's bill balance
    D. A plan for future treatment

18. Your client is a 70-year-old male who lived alone just prior to having a total hip replacement. In order to manage his self-care, the *best* equipment he will need is:
    A. A tea cart with wheels for the kitchen
    B. Dressing stick, sock aid, long-handled shoe horn, bath sponge, and reacher
    C. Tub seat adjusted to his tub at home
    D. Commode for bedside

19. A quadriplegic patient at the C-5 level would have little or no wrist and finger function. The goal of OT would be to enhance wrist extension and tenodesis grasp. How can this *best* be done?
    A. Range finger flexion with wrist flexed
    B. Range finger extension with wrist extended
    C. Range finger flexion with wrist fully extended, finger extension with wrist fully flexed
    D. Makes no difference

20. Licensure for OTs is granted by:
    A. AOTA
    B. NBCOT
    C. A state agency
    D. Both NBCOT and a state agency

21. Many health care programs use management by objective (MBO) plans for the administration of their programs. An MBO plan includes:
    A. A problem-oriented medical record
    B. Overall objective, derived goals, key participants
    C. Subjective, objective, assessment, plan
    D. Indicators, monitors, quality improvement

22. Which of the following behavioral techniques would be *most* appropriate to use with a patient who has agoraphobia?
    A. Habilitation
    B. Extinction
    C. Systematic desensitization
    D. Token economy

23. Brunnstrom was the first to use the treatment of hemiplegia incorporating the use of synergy action. The components of the flexor synergy for the shoulder include:
    A. Scapular adduction, depression, shoulder adduction, and internal rotation
    B. Scapular adduction, elevation, shoulder abduction, and external rotation
    C. Scapular abduction, protraction, shoulder adduction, and internal rotation
    D. Scapular abduction, retraction, and shoulder abduction

24. The components for the flexor synergy of the elbow and forearm include:
    A. Elbow extension and forearm supination
    B. Elbow flexion and forearm supination
    C. Elbow extension and forearm neutral
    D. Elbow extension and forearm pronation

25. Outpatient occupational therapy services are covered under Medicare Part B when:
    A. No OT is available at a local hospital
    B. It's part of an office visit to a physician
    C. Not related to a specific condition
    D. Part A is used up

26. A 60-year-old female client with a history of multiple sclerosis is managed at home with specific adaptations to facilitate function. The patient's family has provided significant care in the area of self-care. You are treating the patient in home care and have noticed she is more withdrawn and recently complained of difficulty swallowing. What is the *best* intervention?
    A. Supportive questioning and explore respite care
    B. Mention your concern to the family
    C. Keep a good log of the patient's responses in therapy
    D. Attribute mood changes and minor problems to the nature of the chronic disease

27. The term that describes principles of occupational therapy practice for individual patients, including guidelines for determining function/dysfunction, motivation, and the change process, is called:
    A. Paradigm
    B. Model
    C. Frame of reference
    D. Therapeutic use of self

28. A lesion in the cerebellum may cause which type of tone?
    A. Rigidity
    B. Hypertonia
    C. Hypotonia
    D. Spasticity

29. Which piece of adaptive equipment is *most* appropriate for a patient with a total knee replacement?
    A. Long-handled shoe horn
    B. Reacher
    C. Sock aid
    D. None of the above

30. Spinal nerves are formed by joining dorsal and ventral roots. They are composed of a mixture of motor, sensory, and autonomic fibers. The ventral root carries which type of information?
    A. Sensory/afferent
    B. Sensory/efferent
    C. Motor/afferent
    D. Motor/efferent

31. The incidence of depression among institutionalized elderly is more prevalent than among their peers living independently in the community. Which of the following statements is the greatest predictor for depression within this long-term elderly population?
    A. Loss of ability to perform ADLs
    B. Late onset of clinical depression
    C. Cognitive impairment
    D. Family history of depression

Use the following information to answer questions 32 through 36: As more occupational therapists work in cardiac rehabilitation, including outpatient or community settings, the understanding of certain concepts is key to good care delivery. For example, the term MET is used in exercise physiology. One MET is equal to 3.5 ml oxygen/kg. This describes the energy required for the average person at rest, such as sitting quietly.

32. On average, self-care activities are at what MET level?
    A. 1
    B. 3
    C. 5
    D. 7

33. Signs of activity-induced cardiovascular dysfunction include all of the following *except:*
    A. Fever
    B. Dyspnea
    C. Altered mental status
    D. Fatigue

34. A cardiac patient in phase 1 in rehabilitation can begin exercise when this occurs:
    A. Generally, 4 days after admission to the hospital
    B. Depression lifts
    C. Free of chest pain
    D. Decrease in anxiety

35. At what point in cardiac rehabilitation does education on diet, stress, medication, and exercise begin?
    A. Phase 1
    B. Phase 2
    C. Phase 3
    D. At discharge

36. The occupational therapist in a cardiac rehabilitation program would consider which goal *most* valuable in the education phase of the patient?
    A. Vocational modification
    B. Energy conservation
    C. Sexual counseling
    D. Relaxation techniques

37. Which reflex is responsible for maintaining normal muscle tone or resistance to movement?
    A. Phasic/dynamic reflex
    B. Static/tonic stretch reflex
    C. Inverse stretch reflex
    D. Withdrawal/flexor reflex

38. According to the National Institute of Mental Health, which of the following statements about suicide is false?
    A. More men than women die by suicide, a ratio of 4:1
    B. Suicide by firearms is the most common method for both men and women
    C. The highest suicide rates are for persons over 65 years of age
    D. Inquiring about suicidal thoughts will implant ideas in people

39. Health care professionals who experience emotional exhaustion, diminished positive feelings toward others, and reduced personal accomplishment may be experiencing what syndrome?
    A. Clinical depression
    B. Dysthymia
    C. Burnout
    D. Stress reaction

40. The OT clinic must have available MSDS (material safety data sheets) on all of the following *except*:
    A. White Out
    B. Theraputty
    C. Soaps
    D. Personal items

41. Often OTAs and OTs work together on the treatment of a particular client. Which is the *best* way to document supervision of the treatment and OTA by the OT?
    A. The OT cosigns the treatment notes in the medical record
    B. The OT keeps a supervision log book when discussing treatment with the OTA
    C. No special documentation is needed because billing is the same for OTAs and OTs
    D. A third party, such as the OT supervisor, documents the collaboration

42. Scapulohumeral rhythm must be taken into account when ranging a shoulder. What is the ratio of scapulo-humeral rhythm?
    A. 1:2 scapula:humerus
    B. 2:1 scapula:humerus
    C. 1:4 scapula:humerus
    D. 4:1 scapula:humerus

43. What pediatric diagnosis is characterized by loss of hand skills developed and abnormal hand movements such as hand wringing and hand washing?
    A. Childhood disintegrative disorder
    B. Childhood schizophrenia
    C. Autism
    D. Rett syndrome

44. What are signs of sensory integrative dysfunction?
    A. Oversensitivity to sound, movement, touch, or visual input
    B. Impulsive, lack of self-control, distraction
    C. Poor self-concept, social problems
    D. All of the above

45. Which is false concerning NDT theory?
    A. Abnormal muscle tone affects muscles but not feeding, speech, or perception
    B. The central nervous system is damaged, resulting in abnormal movements
    C. Change in motor patterns results from the individual feeling more normal movements
    D. An interdisciplinary effort achieves the optimal gains for the individual

46. All of the following techniques are available to the occupational therapist using a cognitive behavioral approach *except*:
    A. Free association
    B. Graded task assignments
    C. Bibliotherapy
    D. Role modeling

47. An activity group in which the client learns group interaction skills through sequential, stage-specific skills is called:
    A. Developmental group
    B. Task-oriented group
    C. Evaluation group
    D. Instrumental group

48. In general, which type of muscle structure provides the greatest ROM?
    A. Fusiform/strap
    B. Spiral
    C. Multipennate
    D. Unipennate

49. According to Yalom, which type of leadership style is *most* useful in the acute inpatient therapy group?
    A. Advisory
    B. Facilitative
    C. Directive
    D. Democratic

50. The occupational therapist has been asked to evaluate a feeding program for a 65-year-old woman with hemiplegia. The patient spilled food because of the inability to adjust her movement when getting food to the mouth. The *most* likely neurobehavioral impairment is:
    A. Ideational apraxia
    B. Motor apraxia
    C. Unilateral body neglect
    D. Perseveration

Section One Answers and Explanations

1. Answer: D
When a patient with a spinal cord injury complains of dizziness, nausea, and is losing consciousness while standing in a standing box, the patient is experiencing postural hypotension. Recline him immediately and get medical assistance if symptoms persist.

2. Answer: B
Work tolerance is the best answer. A, C, and D are performance skills but related to work tolerance.

3. Answer: A
Project level play is for children under 8 years old. B, C, and D are typical of 8-year-olds.

4. Answer: D
The OT does not have to be hospital affiliated, however, A, B, and C are required for Medicare reimbursement.

5. Answer: C
Inflammation of the forearm extensor musculature (ECRB, ECRL, EDC) may result in tennis elbow.

6. Answer: B
Sublimation is the healthy and acceptable rechanneling of the libidinal and aggressive drives into constructive activity. This defense was identified by Anna Freud and remains a basic component to occupational therapy activity. Acting out is often negative and externalizes an unresolved conflict. Identification is a term that incorporates the characteristics of another onto oneself. Regression is going backward to an earlier stage of development.

7. Answer: A
The Practice Framework does not provide any information about fees. B, C, and D are true of *The Practice Framework*.

8. Answer: D
An entry-level OTA is defined as an OTA with less than 1 year of experience. The OTA's work must be supervised by an OT for the first year.

9. Answer: D
Connective tissue disease is not associated with depression, dementia, or psychosis, while Parkinson's, Huntington's, and Wilson's diseases are associated with them.

10. Answer: D
The anterior longitudinal ligament limits extension to protect the vertebral column from excess extension. The posterior longitudinal ligament protects the spine in flexion. Ligamentum flavum is too small, and supraspinatus is a muscle.

11. Answer: D
Abnormal tone, delayed or exaggerated reflexes, and abnormal motor development are all signs of cerebral palsy.

12. Answer: B
Emotional flight is dominated by the sympathetic nervous system.

13. Answer: C
Direct services means the OT is providing face-to-face treatment services.

14. Answer: A
Labile describes abrupt and rapid emotional changes. Anhedonia is the loss of interest and withdrawal from pleasurable activities. Inappropriate affect refers to a mismatch between an emotion and the idea, thought, or speech expressed. Euphoria is the intense feeling of grandeur or happiness.

15. Answer: C
Atrophy is not a symptom of spasticity, while A, B, and D are.

16. Answer: D

An self-employed OT must carry individual coverage.

17. Answer: C

Treatment documentation should not include the patient's bill balance. A, B, and D should be included.

18. Answer: B

The patient will need a dressing stick, sock aid, long-handled shoe horn, bath sponge, and reacher for some time after discharge to achieve independence. A tea cart is not essential, as the patient could slide items on the counter. A tub seat is optional but only if the patient is not safe in the tub. The commode should not be necessary, as most patients at discharge no longer need one; however, a bedside urinal would be adequate if needed or a raised toilet seat could be attached to the home toilet.

19. Answer: C

Tenodesis action is enhanced by shortening the flexor tendons.

20. Answer: C

Licensure is a state responsibility; registration and certification are NBCOT.

21. Answer: B

Overall objective, derived goals, and key participants are unique to MBO plans.

22. Answer: C

Systematic desensitization is an effective treatment for persons with anxiety disorders. A behavioral technique that uses relaxation with an anxiety-producing stimulus will diminish the anxiety response. Habilitation refers to enabling the person to learn a skill he or she has never learned. Extinction is a behavioral approach used to discourage a behavior by ignoring it and reinforcing acceptable ones. Token economy is a reward for a desired behavior.

23. Answer: B

Components of the flexor synergy include scapular adduction, elevation, shoulder abduction, and external rotation. Current theory suggest that evaluation of the flexor synergy is important but questions the usefulness of strengthening these patterns.

24. Answer: B

Components of the flexor synergy include elbow flexion and forearm supination.

25. Answer: B

Outpatient services are covered as part of an office visit to a physician. A, C, and D are not true.

26. Answer: A

Family abuse toward people with disabilities is a significant problem that is often underreported. Supportive questions may clarify this situation and encourage the patient to share her concerns. Dysphagia can be the result of attempted strangulation. B and C are appropriate to typical treatment. D is a weak choice because it ignores the patient's issues.

27. Answer: C

These are defining aspects of frame of reference. A paradigm is a guiding premise and theory that leads to the organization of knowledge, such as the OT profession. A model is a profession's philosophical assumption, ethics, foundation, and domain of concern. Therapeutic use of self is the manner in which the therapist views himself or herself and the impact on one's clients.

28. Answer: C

The cerebellum plays a role in the excitation of gamma motor neurons, which innervate intrafusal fibers within muscles. Damage to the cerebellum causes a decrease in the excitation of gamma motor neurons, which, in turn, leads to a decrease in the sensitivity of the muscle spindles. A decrease in muscle tone results. Hypertonia is an increase in tone. Both rigidity and spasticity are examples of hypertonia.

29. Answer: D

A person with a total knee replacement must learn to bend the knee to increase range of motion. A, B, and C would discourage movement at the knee and therefore are inappropriate.

30. Answer: D

The ventral root carries motor information from the motor cortex out to the muscles. Efferent projections are motor in nature and carry output from a neural structure. Afferent projections are sensory in nature and carry input to a neural structure such as a sensory receptor to the somatosensory lobe.

31. Answer: A

According to Patricia Parmelee, associate director of research at the Philadelphia Geriatric Center, depression is closely linked with physical illness and disability when it causes functional loss. B, C, and D are possible factors in the contribution of depression, however, they do not always lead to depression. Persons experiencing depression in later life seem to be more responsive to treatment.

32. Answer: B

Three times the oxygen used at rest is consumed in self-care activities. Climbing stairs is 5 METs and walking fast is 7 METs.

33. Answer: A

Fever is usually an indicator of infection. B, C, and D are indicators of cardiac dysfunction.

34. Answer: C

The patient must be free of chest pain and should stop exercising at the first sign of pain. B and D are important to address after pain. The patient may need reassurance to the safety of exercise and how he or she is to be monitored. A patient's depression may last up to 6 months.

35. Answer: A

Education begins at phase 1 and includes vocational, family, and sexual issues. Phase 2 continues education and MET level 5 activities. At this level the occupational therapist begins to discuss the return to work and a possible job site evaluation. Phase 3 and outpatient usually coincide.

36. Answer: D

Anxiety and stress are issues of first priority for most patients. Learning to decrease these symptoms is the priority. A, B, and C are also very important but come next in line once the patient is feeling more control.

37. Answer: B

The static/tonic reflex is initiated by a slow stretch of a muscle. This causes stimulation of motor units in the muscle to create resistance. The phasic/dynamic stretch reflex is elicited by rapid muscle stretch and opposes sudden changes in muscle length. The inverse stretch reflex causes a muscle to relax once the maximum tension is reached. The withdrawal/flexor reflex is a response generally initiated by pain or tissue damage. Flexion or withdrawal of the affected body part then occurs.

38. Answer: D

Discussion of feelings regarding suicide with empathy and respect can greatly reduce the distress of a suicidal person and decrease one's sense of isolation. Focusing exclusively about how to commit suicide without considering emotional distress can lead to "copycat" suicides. A, B, and C are all true.

39. Answer: C

During Bailey's investigation in 1990 regarding reasons for OT attrition, 29% of occupational therapists reported "burnout" as their main reason for leaving. This is a type of job stress arising from the social interaction between helper and recipient. Clinical depression is diagnosed with the presence of at least five symptoms including sadness, empty mood, anhedonia, change in sleep and/or appetite, and feelings of worthlessness. Dysthymia is a mild chronic depression lasting 2 or more years. A reaction is a response to a stimulus, while a syndrome is a group of signs/symptoms that characterize a disease process.

40. Answer: D

MSDS are required to protect those exposed to workplace materials. The MSDS provide information in case of an emergency, such as a child eating a piece of Theraputty. MSDS are not required for personal items stored in handbags or lockers, however, safety is always first and an occupational therapist should not use personal items in clinical use without first addressing all safety issues.

41. Answer: B

Cosigning notes is not evidence of supervision. The OT should maintain a separate log book whenever the OTA and OT meet to review cases. C and D are incorrect.

42. Answer: A

In order to provide optimal ROM at the shoulder joint, the scapula must move 1 degree for every 2 degrees of humeral movement. If this does not occur, damage may result. The head of the humerus would not have sufficient space to move in the joint.

43. Answer: D

Rett syndrome is marked by loss of hand skills already acquired in normal development. A, B, and C do not lose hand skills and may or may not have stereotypical hand movements.

44. Answer: D

All are signs including inability to calm self, clumsiness, poor academic achievement, and delay in speech and language skills.

45. Answer: A

According to the NDT Association, abnormal muscle tone and movement affects all function including walking, speech, respiration, feeding, perception, and self-care. B, C, and D are true.

46. Answer: A

Free association is a psychoanalytic technique used by analysts with years of extensive training. All the other cognitive methods are modalities used in OT.

47. Answer: A

Developmental groups were first identified by Anne Mosey and include parallel, project, egocentric-cooperative, cooperative, and mature levels.

48. Answer: A

A muscle fiber can shorten up to one-half its total length. Fusiform or strap muscles are generally longer than other types of muscle and allow the greatest ROM. Spiral and pennate muscle fibers are generally shorter and more numerous, and therefore provide greater strength.

49. Answer: C

Directive leadership means the therapist takes a more active role in the group. The leader provides structure, keeps the group focused, supports members, and ensures efficient use of group time. Acute inpatient group members are usually in crisis and do not have time to reach a mature level. Directive leadership is useful in groups at a low maturity level. Facilitative leadership is effective in groups at a medium to high maturity level. Advisory leadership is effective with highly mature groups. Democratic leadership is a term that correlates with facilitative leadership.

50. Answer: B

Motor apraxia includes the awkward use of tools and poor control of mouth or oral motor control. Ideational apraxia is the misuse of a tool. Unilateral neglect means the patient does not attend to or use her affected arm. Perseveration means the patient is unable to stop movements and may continue to put food in her mouth, resulting in overstuffing.

Section Two

1. Can occupational therapy services be started for a Medicare patient at home?
    A. Only if physical therapy, nursing, or speech is also servicing the patient
    B. Yes, even if OT is alone
    C. Only if two physicians order OT
    D. Yes, if DRGs are still available

2. During an occupational therapy task group, the OT asks a patient to check out his self-perception with others in the group. This thinking process is called:
    A. Autistic thinking
    B. Reality testing
    C. Magical thinking
    D. Illogical thinking

3. Dysdiadochokinesia is a neurological disorder defined as:
    A. A motor problem seen as overshooting or past pointing
    B. A motor problem in which muscles are weak and tire easily
    C. The impaired ability for rapid, repeated alternating movements
    D. Slow, twisting movements

4. The client you are treating is a 60-year-old female with a right CVA. She shows left hemiplegia, severe left homonymous hemianopsia, and left neglect. The *best* approach to facilitate acknowledgment of the left spatial and visual field is:
    A. Remind client to look to the left
    B. Ask family to remind client to look to the left
    C. Ask nursing to remind client to look to the left
    D. Arrange client's environment so it encourages the client to look to the left

5. A hemiplegic patient with shoulder subluxation is *best* treated by:
    A. Wearing a sling for 24 hours a day
    B. Only wearing a sling during gait training
    C. Proper positioning while in bed and in wheelchair
    D. A lap board while in a wheelchair

6. What type of prehension is used to pick up small objects such as pins, nails, or buttons?
    A. Palmar prehension, palmar tripod, or three-jaw chuck
    B. Lateral prehension
    C. Hook grasp
    D. Fingertip prehension

7. When measuring for a wheelchair, what consideration should be made for the seat?
    A. None, seat is standard, no measurements are needed
    B. If doorways in patient's home are narrow, wheelchair seat must be narrow
    C. Seat should be 4 inches wider than patient's widest point across hips or thighs so he or she can move around easier
    D. Seat should be 2 inches wider than patient's widest point across hips or thighs. If braces are worn, width should be increased

8. What fine motor activity is *best* for a 6-year-old child with attention deficit disorder?
   A. Dot-to-dot coloring
   B. Musical instrument such as the piano
   C. Handling a deck of cards
   D. Mazes

9. While performing PROM on your client, you notice spasticity during elbow flexion. Following the spasticity, you notice a sudden relaxation and letting go of tone and full range is achieved. This is called:
   A. Claspknife phenomenon
   B. Clonus
   C. Rigidity
   D. Dystonia

10. A confused head injured patient may ask a lot of questions, often repeating the same question over and over. What is the *best* activity for this patient?
    A. Nothing, the patient is too agitated
    B. Socializing with other patients
    C. Looking at his or her memory book
    D. Playing cards

11. The difference between high technology and low technology is:
    A. Cost
    B. Design
    C. Electronics
    D. Patient diagnosis

12. Which of the following terms describes symptoms caused by abstinence from a substance that the patient has taken over a period of time?
    A. Addiction
    B. Intoxication
    C. Withdrawal
    D. Abuse

13. While assessing the mental status of a patient, the OT could observe which of the following without asking a direct question?
    A. If the patient can subtract 7 from 100 to measure visuospatial ability
    B. If the patient's affect can be described as normal, flat, blunted, constricted
    C. If the patient has visual hallucinations, showing a disturbance in thought process
    D. The patient's mood

14. Residents of a nursing home are often lifetime members of the nursing home community. An OT working in a nursing home must therefore address a resident's needs as if it is his or her home. What activity *best* facilitates fine motor coordination and community development?
    A. Sponsor a float in a community parade, residents can watch
    B. Develop a facility choir and perform for everyone while holding choir music
    C. Make a quilt and raffle it off to purchase something for the facility that members vote on
    D. Build birdhouses and install them outside the windows

15. When working in an activity group with a patient who has AIDS, the occupational therapist should:
    A. Always wear latex gloves
    B. Wash hands before and after treatment
    C. Avoid touching the patient
    D. Always wear a face mask

16. Which early childhood disease is progressive, fatal, and due to fatty fibrous infiltration of muscles?
    A. Postpolio syndrome
    B. Muscular dystrophy
    C. Parkinson's disease
    D. Multiple sclerosis

17. Premature infants usually have mothers who have low socioeconomic status, lack of prenatal care, and poor nutrition. A premature infant is any infant born before:
    A. 37 weeks
    B. 39 weeks
    C. 41 weeks
    D. 43 weeks

18. Vestibular stimulation can be used to increase muscle tone in both adults and children. Always watch the patient for emotional reactions. Spinning should *not* be done with what type of person?
    A. Persons over the age of 50
    B. Persons with poor ROM
    C. Persons prone to seizures
    D. Persons who are 6 feet or over in height

19. Spina bifida is a disorder characterized by failure of the vertebral column to close. Children may have a shunt placed in their head. All of the following are warning signs of a malfunctioning shunt *except*:
    A. Irritability and fussiness
    B. Vomiting
    C. Headache
    D. Wide open eyes, iris is totally visible

20. An upper motor neuron lesion may occur in all of the following *except*:
    A. Brainstem
    B. Spinal cord motor roots
    C. Cranial nerves
    D. Cerebral cortex

21. Occupational therapy services can be paid for under which part(s) of Medicare?
    A. Part A
    B. Part B
    C. Both A and B
    D. Only under supplemental insurance

22. Supervision is considered a professional responsibility and therefore a component of practice. Who is required to have supervision?
    A. All OTAs and entry-level OTs
    B. Entry-level OTAs and OTs
    C. Entry-level OTAs
    D. Entry-level OTs

23. Examination of the efficiency of institutional use and the appropriateness of admissions, services, length of stay, and discharges is called:
    A. Continuous quality assurance
    B. Retrospective analysis
    C. Utilization review
    D. Fee monitoring

24. Which of the following is *not* present at birth?
    A. Moro reflex
    B. Symmetrical postures
    C. Babinski reflex
    D. Impassive facial expression

25. During an intake interview, a patient's ideas constantly shift from one subject to another in an unrelated way. There is no apparent connection to his thoughts. This is called:
    A. Blocking
    B. Perseveration
    C. Flight of ideas
    D. Loose association

26. All of the following are contraindications for aquatic therapy *except*:
    A. Open wound
    B. Decreased cardiovascular endurance
    C. Incontinence
    D. Severe cardiovascular disease

27. When making a forearm trough splint, the splint should be what length of the forearm?
    A. One fourth
    B. One third
    C. One half
    D. Two thirds

28. The *best* activity to assess motor synthesis is:
    A. Playing hopscotch
    B. Guessing an object's name without looking at it
    C. Constructing a three-dimensional box out of paper
    D. Copying a two-dimensional block design

29. All of the following activities are suited to increase spatial relationship awareness *except*:
    A. Making a tall tower of blocks
    B. Doing arithmetic problems
    C. Drawing hands on a clock
    D. Drawing a designated object from memory

30. Your client has a dual diagnosis of hemiplegia and congestive heart failure. You anticipate fluctuating edema in the involved hemiplegic hand. What type of straps should you use on the client's splint?
    A. 1-inch wide webbing with a D ring
    B. 2-inch wide soft Velcro
    C. 4-inch wide Ace wrap
    D. Wide, soft, foam-like strap

31. The ability to derive meaning from an event or experience beyond the tangible aspects of the event itself is known as:
    A. Immediate recall
    B. Abstract thinking
    C. Concentration
    D. Attention

32. In order to increase a patient's compliance with splint usage after discharge, what is the *most* important factor?
    A. Listen to the patient's complaints and adjust splint
    B. Allow the patient to practice donning and doffing the splint
    C. Label the splint
    D. Contrast the colors of the splint and the straps

33. The *best* activity for persons with schizophrenia according to Lorna Jean King is:
    A. A routine exercise program
    B. Country line dancing
    C. Spontaneous movement to music
    D. Tap dancing

34. What neurological pathway in the brainstem is responsible for controlling consciousness and regulating the sleep-wake cycle?
    A. Basal ganglia
    B. Anterior corticospinal tract
    C. Lateral corticospinal tract
    D. Reticular formation

35. Which circuit within the basal ganglia has been implicated to be involved in obsessive-compulsive disorders?
    A. Motor circuit
    B. Oculomotor circuit
    C. Prefrontal association circuit
    D. Limbic circuit

36. An 84-year-old female nursing home resident is 5 years post CVA. Her left hand is in the fisted position and PROM is painful to her. Skin care is a concern. What is the *best* choice for intervention?
    A. None, nothing can be effectively done
    B. Daily soaks to relax the left hand and keep it clean
    C. Resting hand splint
    D. Soft splint

37. Post-traumatic stress disorder is *least* likely to be triggered by:
    A. Job loss
    B. Combat experience
    C. Sexual abuse
    D. Natural catastrophes

38. Intrinsics of the hand include all of the following *except*:
    A. Flexor pollicis longus
    B. Flexor digiti minimi
    C. Flexor pollicis brevis
    D. Abductor pollicis brevis

39. At what age can a child maintain head control when supported in sitting?
    A. 1 month
    B. 2 months
    C. 4 months
    D. 5 months

40. A child of 2 to 3 years old who grabs a chunky crayon with his fingers while his wrist is pronated is showing what type of grasp?
    A. Mature dynamic tripod
    B. Less mature static tripod
    C. Immature pronated grasp
    D. Power grasp

41. All of the following are spinal cord level reflexes *except*:
    A. Rooting, sucking
    B. Flexor withdrawal, placing
    C. Stepping, galant
    D. Asymmetric tonic neck reflex, symmetric tonic neck reflex

42. The *most* common classification of cerebral palsy is:
    A. Spasticity
    B. Athetosis
    C. Flaccid/atonia
    D. Mixed

43. Developmental tasks of a person in later adulthood include all of the following *except:*
    A. Acceptance of one's self and life
    B. Acceptance of one's ethnic origin and identity
    C. Acceptance of one's mortality
    D. Acceptance of one's sexual identity

44. Tetraplegia is a term that indicates:
    A. The involvement of only the hands in plegia
    B. The involvement of only the lower extremities
    C. The involvement of only one side
    D. The involvement of four limbs

45. Post-polio syndrome can be associated with all of the following *except:*
    A. Weakness
    B. Fatigue
    C. Rapid onset of symptoms
    D. Chronic overuse resulting in limb pain

46. Pervasive development disorders include all of the following *except:*
    A. Autism
    B. Asperger's disorder
    C. Rett syndrome
    D. Childhood schizophrenia

47. A child in a full inclusion classroom requires staff and parent education to succeed. The role of the occupational therapist includes all of the following *except:*
    A. Educate the teacher on body mechanics so the teacher does not hurt her back when moving the child
    B. Educate the parents on techniques to maintain performance in the classroom
    C. Advise the parents on medical procedures that can enhance classroom performance
    D. Educate the teacher's aide to optimum classroom positioning and seating for the child

48. A 17-year-old young man with autism has been successful in all his occupational therapy treatments except shaving. His female classroom teacher reports some peers are teasing him about his "5 o'clock shadow." The teenager lives at home with his single mother and two younger sisters. The mother is frustrated because she has to nag the teen to get him to shave in the morning. As the school-based consulting OT, what is the *best* option for treatment:
    A. Have the teen wait to shave until he gets to school and then have his teacher supervise
    B. Allow the teen's beard to grow in and not shave at all
    C. Start a shaving group with all the young men in the teen's classroom
    D. Arrange a male teen volunteer to role model shaving with the young man

49. All of the following are foundations of the spatiotemporal adaptation frame of reference *except:*
    A. Adaptation occurs with interaction of the individual and environment over time and space
    B. Spatiotemporal stress is both positive and negative
    C. Processing develops from reflex to motor planning
    D. Handling and positioning are used with inhibiting techniques

50. Sensory integration development continues throughout life but is generally complete by what age?
    A. 1 to 3 years of age
    B. 4 to 5 years of age
    C. 8 to 10 years of age
    D. 14 to 18 years of age

Section Two Answers and Explanations

1. Answer: A

At the time of the printing of this book, physical therapy, nursing, or speech also had to service the home care patient before the OT could initiate service. AOTA is working to change this policy.

2. Answer: B

Reality testing is the process of evaluating and judging one's external environment in an objective manner. Autistic thinking refers to a preoccupation with one's inner world. Magical thinking is when thoughts, words, or actions are believed to assume power. Illogical thinking is contradicting and erroneous.

3. Answer: C

Dysdiadochokinesia is impaired alternating movement. Overshooting is dysmetria, weak muscles is asthenia, and slow, twisting movements is athetosis.

4. Answer: D

All are good choices, but arranging the client's environment to encourage looking to the left is best. This should be done as long as the patient is cognitively aware of the neglect. If the patient is not cognitively aware of the left, visitors or other stimulus approaching from the left may scare her. Remind family and staff to announce their presence as they enter.

5. Answer: C

Subluxation itself is not painful but poor handling is. Transfers and PROM will potentially cause soft tissue damage. Pay special attention in handling and in scapula mobilization. Slings are not always helpful and should not be used 24 hours per day. A lap board may be helpful when the patient is in a wheelchair but does not address the global issue.

6. Answer: D

Fingertip prehension requires fine motor coordination. It allows one to sew, snap, or button. Palmar prehension involves three fingers for writing or eating. Lateral prehension is used when turning a key. It generally involves the thumb. Hook prehension is thumbless and is used when carrying a handle, case, or heavy object.

7. Answer: D

Two inches wider than the user is correct. One size does not fit all and too much padding or room can cause sores.

8. Answer: A

Although all activities are fine motor, age and diagnosis must be considered. B, C, and D may be too advanced for this child.

9. Answer: A

Continued passive stretching of spastic muscle may produce a sudden letting go relaxation. Claspknife phenomenon may be seen in neurological disorders of upper motor neuron lesions. Clonus is a spasmodic alteration of muscle contraction and relaxation. Rigidity is relatively constant hypertonicity. Dystonia is a tone disorder resulting in slow movement or decreased tone.

10. Answer: C

The OT could make a memory book for the patient that includes answers to common questions like, "Where am I?" Include family pictures and reality orientation information. Keep the book simple to reduce agitation and light in case the patient should throw it. Having the patient play cards or socialize with others may be too much stimulation. Doing nothing is likely to get the patient more agitated.

11. Answer: C

The difference between high and low technology is electronics.

12. Answer: C

Withdrawal is a group of symptoms that appears within hours to 1 week of abstinence from a substance. Examples include delirium, tremors, seizures, psychosis, perceptual disturbances, irritability, and gastrointestinal and sympathetic hyperactivity. Addiction refers to a behavior and physical dependence, not a symptom. Intoxication is a state of progressive deterioration ranging from exhilaration to stupefaction caused by ingesting substances. Abuse refers to a maladaptive pattern leading to clinically significant impairment or distress.

13. Answer: B

The patient's affect shows his or her emotional responsiveness. This may affect the data collected during the rest of the intake. Asking the patient to subtract 7 from 100 is measuring attention and knowledge. Hallucinations are disturbances in perception. Mood is a pervasive, sustained emotion reported by the patient.

14. Answer: C

All the activities encourage either community involvement or fine motor skills, but only the quilt fundraiser provides both.

15. Answer: B

The OT should use universal precautions with all patients whether they have AIDS or not. The person with AIDS is at greater risk of catching a disease from the therapist. Staff should wash their hands before and after all treatments. The OT needs to wear a mask only if he or she has a cold. Latex gloves are only needed if there is a risk of contact with bodily fluids.

16. Answer: B

Only muscular dystrophy is an early childhood, progressive, and fatal disease due to fatty infiltration of the muscles. Post-polio syndrome is weakened musculature following poliomyelitis. Parkinson's is a slow, progressive disease with onset after age 40. Multiple sclerosis is due to a demyelination of the nerves.

17. Answer: A

A premature infant is any infant born before 37 weeks.

18. Answer: C

Spinning is contraindicated for people prone to seizures. The patient may not be able to tolerate the vestibular input, thereby triggering a seizure.

19. Answer: D

Irritability, vomiting, headaches, and "setting sun" eyes are all symptoms of a malfunctioning shunt. "Setting sun" eyes are partially visible irises.

20. Answer: B

The anterior motor roots within the spinal cord are considered lower motor neuron. The CNS includes the brainstem, cranial nerves, and the cerebral cortex.

21. Answer: C

Occupational therapy can be paid for under both Parts A and B of Medicare.

22. Answer: C

Entry-level OTAs are required to have supervision by OTs for the first year. All OT personnel should have supervision as needed to match their level of competence.

23. Answer: C

Utilization review is an internal management review on how resources are utilized.

24. Answer: B

Symmetrical postures predominate at 16 weeks. The startle reflex is present at birth when flexion of the extremities occurs when scared. Babinski can be induced by stroking the sole of the foot and the big toe rises. This is normal until age 1, but after the toe should plantar flex. Impassive facial expressions are typical social behavior of an infant under 4 weeks of age.

25. Answer: D

Loose associations are a disturbance of thought. In severe cases, the patient may become incoherent. Blocking refers to abrupt interruptions in thinking. Perseveration refers to persistent responses often found in cognitive disorders. Flight of ideas refers to rapid thinking with shifting in ideas that are slightly connected.

26. Answer: B

A person with decreased cardiovascular endurance may benefit from aquatic therapy. A, C, and D do not indicate readiness.

27. Answer: D

Two thirds length allows full elbow motion and distributes weight over the length. This splint is a first-class lever with the pivot point or fulcrum at the wrist. The long trough distributes the weight of the hand and acts as a counter-balance. A, B, and C are too short.

28. Answer: A

Hopscotch involves motor synthesis. Answer B is tactile perception, C is cognitive problem solving, and D is visual motor synthesis.

29. Answer: D

Drawing from memory is a visual motor synthesis activity.

30. Answer: D

Wide, soft, foam-like strap is the best choice because it allows for slight fluctuations in edema. A, B, and C are less favorable.

31. Answer: B

Ability to abstract is to take an event such as a picnic and value the friendship of the people you are with as well as the food. Immediate recall is remembering information within 1 minute. Concentration is the ability to maintain attention for longer periods to complete a task. Attention is the ability of the CNS to focus on relevant stimuli while screening out the irrelevant.

32. Answer: A

Compliance is enhanced if the therapist has listened to the patient's issues concerning feel and fit. B, C, and D are also valuable to apply in treatment.

33. Answer: C

Lorna Jean King believed that persons with schizophrenia have ineffective proprioceptive feedback mechanisms with an underactive vestibular regulating system. Activities should be non-cortical and pleasurable, since thinking about movements tends to slow down a person. A, B, and D all require attention to the movement patterns.

34. Answer: D

The reticular formation dispersed throughout the brainstem is responsible. The basal ganglia are not located in the brainstem. Although the anterior and lateral corticospinal tracts do pass through the brainstem, they are primarily involved in motor control.

35. Answer: C

The prefrontal association circuit is involved in cognitive processing, which includes attention switching. This circuit is believed to be affected in patients who are unable to control ritualistic and repetitive behaviors. The motor circuit aids in making movements automatic and coordinated and is believed to be involved in Parkinson's disorder. The oculomotor circuit plays a role in the control of eye movements and is believed to be involved in Parkinson's disorder and Huntington's disease. The limbic circuit plays a role in emotions and motivation and is believed to be involved in behaviors associated with Tourette's syndrome.

36. Answer: D

A soft splint, such as a palm protector, places joints in submaximum extension. This allows for adequate skin hygiene. Answer A is not true as options are available. Nursing can provide warm soaks. The resting hand splint is too rigid and likely painful for this particular resident.

37. Answer: A

Emotional stress of serious magnitude that is traumatic for almost everyone contributes to the development of PTSD. Recent research has placed greater emphasis on a person's subjective response to trauma than on the severity of the stress itself. A majority of people do not develop PTSD even when faced with overwhelming trauma.

38. Answer: A

The flexor pollicis longus originates on the body of the radius and inserts on the base of the distal phalanx of digit 1. Therefore, the muscle belly is located within the forearm and not the hand. B, C, and D all have muscle bellies located in the hand.

39. Answer: B

A child can maintain head control while supported at 2 months. At 1 month the child can move his or her head slightly while in prone. At 4 to 5 months the child can hold his or her chest off the floor while in prone.

40. Answer: C

A mature dynamic tripod grasp is typical of a 5- to 6-year-old. A less mature static tripod is used by a 3- to 4-year-old and the hand moves instead of the fingers during writing. A power grasp is used by a 1-year-old and is fisted with the wrist flexed.

41. Answer: D

ATNR and STNR are brainstem level reflexes.

42. Answer: A

Spasticity is most common and includes hyperactive deep tendon reflexes. Athetosis has varying muscle tone, atonia is low tone, and mixed is usually spastic with athetosis.

43. Answer: D

Acceptance of one's sexual identity is a developmental task of later adolescence (18 to 22 years).

44. Answer: D

The American Spinal Cord Injury Association states that tetraplegia is the preferred term to indicate impairment or loss of motor and/or sensory function at the cervical level.

45. Answer: C

PPS has a slow onset appearing decades after the acute onset of polio or after decades of stable functioning. A, B, and D are classic signs of PPS.

46. Answer: D

Pervasive developmental disorders are distinct from schizophrenia, although children with PPD may occasionally develop schizophrenia later in life.

47. Answer: C

The occupational therapist does not advise about medical procedures but may encourage the parent to ask the child's medical staff for advice.

48. Answer: D

As a consultant, you are advising the teacher and parent. Having the teenager wait until school to shave puts shaving out of the home and into an inappropriate site. Starting a shaving group would only be appropriate if everyone else in the class needed instruction but this is not the case. Currently, the young man has no male role models as everyone around him of importance is female. A male teenager volunteer could be advised to role model shaving and offer words of encouragement. An electric shaver could provide added safety.

49. Answer: D

Handling, positioning, and inhibiting techniques are NDT terms. NDT techniques can be used along with spatiotemporal frame of reference but are not foundations as are A, B, and C.

50. Answer: C

Even older adults can improve sensory integration and being active through life can facilitate this, however, basic sensory integration development is generally developed by age 8 to 10.

Section Three

1. What grasp pattern uses both thumb and fingers to hold an object against the palm?
   A. Lateral or key grasp
   B. Radial digit grasp
   C. Pad to pad grasp
   D. Cylindrical grasp

2. If you were asked to perform a neurological examination on a 40-year-old client with a CVA, what should you include in the evaluation?
   A. Coordination evaluation
   B. Apraxia evaluation
   C. Cognitive testing
   D. Perceptual evaluation

3. An entry-level OTA has the necessary knowledge to perform what type of evaluations?
   A. Perceptual
   B. Cognitive
   C. ADL
   D. Sensory motor

4. Medicare Part A pays for all *except*:
   A. Hospital inpatient stay
   B. Physician outpatient visits
   C. Skilled nursing facility
   D. Home and hospice care

5. Which assessment is *best* to evaluate motor skills in an adult?
   A. Adult Activity Inventory
   B. Purdue Pegboard
   C. Comprehensive Occupational Therapy Evaluation (COTE)
   D. Southern California Sensory Integration Tests (SCSIT)

6. ADA has had sweeping reforms in barrier-free designs. When planning the floor space of any department, what is the minimum width of a door frame?
   A. 28 inches
   B. 30 inches
   C. 32 inches
   D. 36 inches

7. Occupational therapy managers should develop departmental policies for all of the following reasons *except*:
   A. Policies clarify prohibited behaviors
   B. Policies negate the code of ethics
   C. Policies are guides to thinking and action
   D. Policies suggest courses of action

8. What activity is *best* to encourage co-contraction in children with low tone?
    A. Playing "Statue"
    B. Going through an obstacle course
    C. Pretending to ice skate around the room
    D. Finger painting

9. A life skills management group to increase functional skills would include all of the following *except*:
    A. Increasing conversations
    B. Food preparation
    C. Problem solving
    D. Money management

10. SOAP notes are sometimes used for documentation. In what section would the patient's comments during treatment go?
    A. Subjective (S)
    B. Objective (O)
    C. Assessment (A)
    D. Plan (P)

11. Where would you locate the acromion process?
    A. Humerus
    B. Clavicle
    C. Scapula
    D. Vertebrae

12. A deformity in which the finger is positioned in extreme PIP flexion and DIP hyperextension is called:
    A. Ulnar deviation
    B. Boutonniere
    C. Swan neck
    D. Intrinsic plus

13. Your client is a 75-year-old female who has significant hyposensitivity in the left arm following a right CVA. The *most* important intervention for this client would be:
    A. Sensory re-education
    B. Safety and compensation instruction
    C. Motor and movement therapy of the left UE
    D. Self-care instructions with emphasis on the non-involved limb

14. What factor is *most* important in OT staff retention?
    A. High salaries
    B. Job satisfaction
    C. Continuing education opportunities
    D. Health insurance benefits

15. Research in occupational therapy is:
    A. Well-developed and complete
    B. Usually done with other disciplines
    C. In the early stages of growth and development
    D. Of little value because it is statistical in nature

16. Your client is a 6-year-old boy who is highly distractible. You have designed a very structured program aimed at providing a successful experience for the patient. Your environment should be:

    A. Bright colors with several choices of toys for fine motor skill development

    B. Distracting and competitive stimuli are low

    C. A simulated classroom

    D. No particular environmental factors need to be addressed due to the structured program

17. Capital expenses of an occupational therapy program might include:

    A. Land and buildings

    B. Supplies

    C. Equipment under $500.00

    D. OT staff salaries

18. The unconscious forgetting of an idea that is anxiety producing and unacceptable to the person in some way is known as:

    A. Dementia

    B. Repression

    C. Impaired judgment

    D. Regression

19. Which of the following statements is *not* true about psychotropic medication?

    A. Imipramine was the first tricyclic antidepressant to be discovered

    B. Thorazine signaled the beginning of modern psychopharmacology for antipsychotic medication

    C. Prozac is a relatively safe drug for treating schizophrenia

    D. Ritalin is effective in treating attention deficit disorder

20. Doorknobs should be placed at what height from the floor to allow for accessibility for people in wheelchairs?

    A. 28 inches

    B. 30 inches

    C. 32 inches

    D. 36 inches

21. The format for documentation is largely:

    A. Decided by management at the facility

    B. Agreed upon by majority rule within the OT department

    C. Outlined by regulation or law

    D. Developed by faculty from OT schools

22. Certification of an OTA is granted by:

    A. AOTA, AMA, and APA jointly

    B. OTA's own association

    C. State certification boards

    D. NBCOT

23. Your client is a 4-year-old girl with cerebral palsy and very low tone. When she is positioned in her customized wheelchair, her head is forward and she cannot maintain the vertical position. What is the *best* intervention?

    A. Recline the wheelchair so gravity will pull her head into neutral

    B. Give verbal commands to pull up her head

    C. Present an object in her visual field to elicit extension through eye tracking

    D. Use a soft cervical collar or molded neck collar to increase head control

24. The mother of a 5-year-old child with developmental delays tells you that she is unable to do his home care program because she is "too busy." You suspect that there might be other reasons. What should you do *first*?

    A. Emphasize the importance of the home program

    B. Discontinue the program and see the client in the clinic again

    C. Talk to the mother about problems she is facing

    D. Provide more information on how to make the home program easier

25. MMT is a valuable test of muscle power. It can also provide additional information on all of the following *except*:

    A. Resistance muscles can tolerate

    B. Muscle endurance

    C. ROM through which joints pass

    D. Gains or losses in strength

26. What disorder is characterized by the presence of one or more neurological symptoms such as paralysis, blindness, and/or paresis; has no known neurological or medical base; and psychological factors are associated with the initiation or exacerbation of symptoms?

    A. Hypochondriasis

    B. Korsakoff's syndrome

    C. Conversion disorder

    D. Dissociative identity disorder

27. Myopathies are a group of muscle diseases whose common principle symptom is generally proximal weakness. Which activity, if performed suboptimally, could indicate a myopathy?

    A. Eating a bowl of soup

    B. Climbing stairs

    C. Brushing teeth

    D. Donning pants

28. A person with a spinal cord injury who complains of dizziness and feels faint may be experiencing:

    A. Autonomic dysreflexia

    B. Pulmonary emboli

    C. Orthostatic hypotension

    D. Abdominal distention

29. Pressure ulcers are a concern in chronic rehabilitation. The *most* important consideration in the management of pressure ulcers is:

    A. Early detection

    B. Prevention

    C. Understanding potential signs

    D. Understanding friction force and support surfaces

30. Deep vein thrombi can result from all conditions *except*:
    A. Myocardial infarction
    B. Prolonged immobilization
    C. CVA/stroke
    D. Reflex sympathetic dystrophy

31. A person with a spinal cord injury who has active wrist extension and tenodesis function is at what level?
    A. C-4
    B. C-5
    C. C-6
    D. C-9

32. A client with a C-5 spinal cord injury is ready to address self-feeding. What piece of equipment would the client benefit *most* from?
    A. Mobile arm support
    B. Universal cuff
    C. Electric wheelchair
    D. Scoop dish

33. In a pediatric population, what type of equipment is *most* effective for vestibular treatment?
    A. Suspended equipment
    B. ADL equipment
    C. Computer equipment
    D. Pen and paper tasks in a classroom

34. A blind or visually impaired person may have some sight. All of the following can assist the individual in his or her home environment *except*:
    A. Contrasting scatter rugs by the doors
    B. A dark placemat or cup on a light surface
    C. Stair risers painted in a contrasting color
    D. White tape to mark a dark object

35. When an elderly person has lost all vision, all of the following are helpful *except*:
    A. Textured surfaces to indicate the top and bottom of stairs
    B. Safety pins in different arrangements to mark clothes
    C. Textured doorknobs to mark exits
    D. Labels or signs in Braille

36. As part of managed health care, cross training is used. This involves:
    A. OTs cotreating the patient at the same time with a PT
    B. Many disciplines being able to meet the client's basic needs
    C. OTs continuing their education to avoid being laid off
    D. OTs being physically fit so they work at maximum efficiency

37. Critical paths are:
    A. Planned treatment schedules based on effective treatment approaches
    B. An environmental simulation that has different textures
    C. A warning that the patient may have an infectious disease
    D. Important documentation that is found in the front of the medical record

38. When should discharge plans begin?
    A. At admission
    B. Once the patient is out of the critical care unit
    C. When rehabilitation begins
    D. At least 1 week before the patient is ready for discharge

39. When a patient is frightened to transfer out of bed and into a wheelchair, the occupational therapist should do all of the following *except:*
    A. Use a firm touch and hurried motions to make the transfer as quick as possible
    B. Tell the patient what you intend to do and how you will do it
    C. Answer "I can't" with "Yes, you can, and I will help you"
    D. Instruct one step at a time

40. Basic body mechanics assist both the patient and the therapist. All of the following are good body mechanics *except:*
    A. When possible push, pull, or slide an object rather than pick it up
    B. Slight body twisting will provide more lift when picking up a heavy object
    C. Maintain your center of gravity (COG) close to the COG of the object you are holding
    D. Widen your base of support to stabilize your vertical gravity line

41. The *best* way to clean a wheelchair after it has been exposed to rain or snow is:
    A. Hose it down with clean water
    B. Let it air dry
    C. Use a light oil on the cross-brace center pin
    D. Wipe it dry with a cloth using a metal cleaner if needed

42. Severe swallowing disorders are associated with:
    A. High risk of aspiration
    B. Olfactory changes
    C. Nasal tumors
    D. Poor oral hygiene

43. A person with Alzheimer's disease who is unable to manage bathing but is still able to choose the proper clothing for the season might indicate a differential diagnosis of:
    A. Arthritis
    B. Schizophrenia
    C. Myocardial infarction
    D. Multiple sclerosis

44. Signs of extrapyramidal reactions include all of the following *except*:
    A. Lip puckering or smacking
    B. Inability to sustain tongue movement
    C. Frowning, blinking, smiling, or grimacing
    D. Arms rapidly moving without objective or slow athetoid movements

45. When teaching elderly clients about their medication routine, keep information short and to the point, be concrete about the time the medication should be taken, provide written directions at the end of the session, and:
    A. Use the words "drugs" or "pills" instead of the word "medicine"
    B. Ask the client to repeat information back to you
    C. Use technical words as well as common language
    D. Change all bottles to easy-open caps

46. Which of the following alternatives to restraints for the confused elderly is *not* effective?
    A. Structured, predictable routine
    B. Several activities to choose from
    C. Validate feelings; if resident is looking for mother, attend to the feelings behind it
    D. Place names and pictures on door

47. Which of the following alternatives to restraints for the wandering elderly is *not* effective?
    A. Opportunity for exercise
    B. Put bells on their shoes
    C. Safe, closed area outside or inside
    D. Identity bracelet

48. Mildred Ross' five-stage integrative group therapy includes orientation, movement activities, visual perceptual motor activities, cognitive activities, and:
    A. Closure activities to establish environmental trust
    B. Sensory integration activities
    C. Memory activities to stimulate abstract thinking
    D. Exercise to facilitate muscle tone

49. Activities that are alerting to the sensory integrative systems include all of the following *except*:
    A. Fast, loud music of variable intensity
    B. Swinging or sustained movements
    C. Light touch, whisking, brushing movements
    D. Increased muscle activities

50. Which assessment can be used in a geriatric setting, providing information on a patient's independent activities of daily living and effective outcome measures as well?
    A. Kohlman Evaluation of Living Skills
    B. Barthel Index
    C. First STEP
    D. Peabody Developmental Motor Scales

Section Three Answers and Explanations

1. Answer: D
Cylindrical grasp is correct. All the others are types of pinch.

2. Answer: A
A neurological evaluation would always include a review of the gross motor and fine motor coordination. B, C, and D are appropriate for follow-up based on initial neurological screening.

3. Answer: C
An entry-level OTA can complete an ADL evaluation and can assist in perceptual, cognitive, and sensory motor evaluations.

4. Answer: B
Medicare Part A pays for inpatient care and does not cover outpatient visits.

5. Answer: B
The Purdue Pegboard is a test of motor skills. The Adult Activity Inventory is a leisure skills evaluation. The COTE is a behaviorally based test of general performance. The SCSIT is a pediatric test of sensory integration.

6. Answer: C
The width of the door opening should be a minimum of 32 inches.

7. Answer: B
The code of ethics cannot be altered.

8. Answer: A
Co-contraction requires both extensor and flexor muscles to be active. This means that the child must stay still, like in the game "Statue." B, C, and D are activities that work on gross motor skills and require movement.

9. Answer: C
Problem solving is considered a cognitive skill. A, B, and D are all skills included in life management and daily living.

10. Answer: A
Subjective data are any data that the patient told the therapist. Objective data are fact-based from the OT.

11. Answer: C
The acromion process is found on the posterior lateral aspect of the scapula. Palpated to assess subluxation, it is also the axis of goniometry.

12. Answer: B
Boutonniere is described. Ulnar deviation is MCP deviation. Swan neck is PIP extension and DIP flexion. Intrinsic is a soft tissue test.

13. Answer: B
Safety is the first concern to prevent patient injury such as bumping or burning the involved limb. The patient must be taught compensation techniques for the sensory loss. Sensory re-education is a low priority. Spontaneous recovery may occur. Sensory loss does result in decreased motor function. The therapist should work on increasing movement, considering safety first. Self-care would follow compensation techniques. The patient would need to work safely in her environment.

14. Answer: B
Job satisfaction is the number one reason why staff stay in one facility. Salaries, benefits, and education, while important, fall below satisfaction.

15. Answer: C

Although great gains have been made lately, research in OT is still considered to be in its infancy when compared to other arts and sciences. Lack of research can lead to some people thinking of occupational therapy as a second-class science. For this reason, AOTF makes research a top priority.

16. Answer: B

A client with high distractibility requires an environment with low stimuli to focus on a task. A and C are inappropriate. D is not true.

17. Answer: A

Capital expenses are major costs such as land and buildings. Supplies and equipment are direct costs if used for treatment, indirect if used as office supplies. OT staff salaries vary if direct patient care or management.

18. Answer: B

Repression is unconscious forgetting as a means of coping. Dementia refers to organic deterioration of intellectual functioning. Impaired judgment refers to the inability to assess a situation correctly and act. Regression refers to the returning to an earlier level of functioning.

19. Answer: C

Prozac has promising effects for depression, obsessive-compulsive disorder, and bulimia. Prozac is not an antipsychotic drug. All the other answers are true.

20. Answer: D

Doorknobs should be located 36 inches from the floor to allow for access for a person using a wheelchair.

21. Answer: C

Documentation must comply with regulation and laws first. Management, OT staff, and, at times, faculty can provide suggestions within the regulations.

22. Answer: D

Only NBCOT offers certification for OTAs.

23. Answer: D

The patient needs to feel the value of a vertical position and to gain head control but still needs support in the wheelchair. If tipped back, she will never be upright. This does not treat the problem. Verbal commands will only lead to frustration of both patient and therapist. Using an object can help develop strength but cannot be used continuously.

24. Answer: C

Until you speak with the mother, you will not know what the problem is. The program may be too difficult or the mother may be overwhelmed with the responsibility. When treating a child with severe disabilities, the OT is often treating the whole family. Take time to meet with the mother privately and provide her with the support she needs.

25. Answer: B

Muscle endurance (defined as how many times the muscle can contract) is not determined by MMT. Resistance, ROM, and strength gains/losses can all be measured with MMT.

26. Answer: C

These are typical signs of conversion disorder. Hypochondriasis is a preoccupation with disease that is unrealistic or inaccurate in relation to actual physical symptoms. Korsakoff's syndrome is an amnestic disorder caused by thiamine deficiency not uncommon in persons with chronic alcohol abuse or poor nutritional habits. Dissociative identity disorder is also known as multiple personality and is caused by a severe traumatic event.

27. Answer: B

Weakness in the proximal hip musculature makes climbing stairs difficult for a person with myopathy. The client could lean forward to support himself or herself and continue to use distal function for A and C. Donning pants could be achieved by sitting.

28. Answer: C

The client cannot tolerate an upright position and may require a graded program in a reclining back wheelchair. Autonomic dysreflexia is a life-threatening rise in blood pressure with headache and coma. Death can occur if untreated. A pulmonary emboli is also life-threatening and includes respiratory distress. Answer D is observable in some cases.

29. Answer: B

All items are important but prevention is key.

30. Answer: D

Stroke, immobilization, and MI are all at risk for DVT. Fifty percent of all people with CVA experience DVT. The lower extremities should be evaluated daily for discoloration, edema, and pain. RSD is not associated with DVT.

31. Answer: C

C-6 innervates extensor carpi radialis longus and brevis. C-5 has elbow flexors and limited distal function. C-4 has absence of arm function.

32. Answer: B

A mobile arm support may assist the client in holding up his or her arm, but most clients prefer to use as little equipment as possible. A scoop dish may be helpful, but the universal cuff is necessary because the client will not have hand function. The electric wheelchair is not necessary for feeding, but the client should be able to use a lightweight manual chair.

33. Answer: A

Suspended equipment, such as swings, is effective in treating vestibular disorders.

34. Answer: A

Scatter rugs are dangerous to everyone. They are the cause of many home accidents, particularly to those with visual or mobility issues. Scatter rugs are often the cause of falls in the elderly.

35. Answer: D

Often older people lose their sight and do not want to learn Braille. The elderly usually prefer to adjust their environment with cues such as a rubber band on the orange juice but not on the milk.

36. Answer: B

Cross training means that several disciplines can provide for a patient's basic needs. For example, the psychologist can assist the client with using the bathroom, the occupational therapist can assist the client with ambulation.

37. Answer: A

Critical paths or pathways are predetermined treatment plans for routine treatments. For example, a rehabilitation program may have a critical path for a person with a total hip replacement that lays out what is to be reached at days 1, 3, and 5 of rehabilitation. Although critical paths may seem like cookie cutter treatment plans, they are effective in typical patient progress and reduce documentation needs on the occupational therapist.

38. Answer: A

Discharge plans are most effective when begun at admission. This is true in both medical and psychiatric admissions and provides a focus for the treatment plan.

39. Answer: A

Use of a gentle touch and unhurried motions will reassure the patient.

40. Answer: B
Avoid twisting your body for all lifts.

41. Answer: D
Do not hose a wheelchair with water or let it air dry. Wipe it clean with a metal cleaner available in the car care section of department stores. Do not use a light oil on any part of the wheelchair as it will collect dirt. Use a molybdenum-based grease on the cross-brace every 6 months. Educate your patients to follow the owner's manual.

42. Answer: A
Aspiration is life-threatening and occurs when food passes through the larynx and into the lungs. Up to 60% of a nursing home population may need a swallowing program.

43. Answer: A
People with arthritis often have problems with bathing and these signs should not be confused with the dementia. B, C, and D have issues with ADLs in general, not just bathing.

44. Answer: B
All are signs of extrapyramidal syndrome (EPS) except inability to sustain tongue movements. EPS includes increased movement in tongue, both in and out of the mouth. In addition, EPS can include jaw biting, clenching, chewing, or mouth opening.

45. Answer: B
Have client repeat information back by asking: "We have covered a lot of information today. Can you summarize all the important information for me?" Always use the word medicine instead of pills or drugs. Avoid technical words altogether and never change the medication bottles. If the client is having a hard time with the bottles, encourage the client to ask the pharmacist to change the bottles for him or her.

46. Answer: B
Elderly who are cognitively impaired, such as dementia patients, do well in structured programs with activities, however, too many choices can be confusing. Validating feelings can greatly reduce anxiety. Names and pictures on doors help the resident find his or her room.

47. Answer: B
Wandering elderly are often confused as well. Bells on their shoes may act as an alarm but not likely. A safe environment inside and closed outside allows wandering without danger.

48. Answer: A
Closure activities is the last stage on the five-stage group. This includes closing on a positive note, asserting internal control, expressing pleasure, and leaving appropriately.

49. Answer: B
Mildred Ross describes this as a calming activity.

50. Answer: B
Although the KELS measures ADLs, it is a test developed to use once and predict ability to live independently. C and D are pediatric assessments. The Barthel can be used for functional outcome measures as well as patient evaluation.

Section Four

1. What reflex is developmentally appropriate until age 5 months, vital for newborns, and can be seen when the corner of the infant's mouth is stroked?

    A. Grasp reflex

    B. Galant reflex

    C. Primary righting action

    D. Rooting reflex

2. An individual member of AOTA in good standing is one who has done all of the following *except*:

    A. Paid membership fees

    B. Upheld the standards and ethics of the association

    C. Met the qualifications for membership

    D. Made a significant contribution to the profession

Use the following information to answer questions 3 and 4: During an occupational therapy task group, you observe your patient's cognitive abilities. George is able to complete a simple three-step craft project with visual cueing from the occupational therapist at each step. While disregarding the written directions, George uses the sample project as a guide. His attention span is intact for 45 minutes.

3. According to Claudia Allen, at what level is your patient performing?

    A. Level 3, manual

    B. Level 4, goal-directed

    C. Level 5, exploratory

    D. Level 6, planned

4. According to Allen, besides a simple craft project, what other activity would be *best* for George to work on cognitive functioning?

    A. Playing the game "Simon Says"

    B. Making a sandwich

    C. Budgeting for 1 day

    D. Making a model airplane that snaps together

5. When determining staff requirements for a new occupational therapy department, the *most* important factor to consider is:

    A. Patient load requirements

    B. Size of the space where OT will be housed

    C. The number of physical therapists

    D. Type of funding available

6. Membership to AOTA is open to:

    A. Occupational therapy students

    B. OTs

    C. OTAs

    D. All of the above

7. Performance in areas of occupation in *The Practice Framework* include:
   A. Self-care
   B. Work
   C. Play/leisure
   D. All of the above

8. You have just completed an ADL evaluation on a 65-year-old female. She had a right CVA in the nondominant hemisphere parietal lobe. During the evaluation you noticed the patient dressed the unaffected limb but did not dress the affected limb. This is an indication of:
   A. Motor apraxia
   B. Ideational apraxia
   C. Unilateral body neglect
   D. Astereognosis

9. Manual muscle testing should be performed on all patients *except*:
   A. C-4 spinal cord injury
   B. Multiple sclerosis
   C. Spastic hemiplegia CVA
   D. Non-acute rheumatoid arthritis

Use the following information to answer questions 10 and 11: Your client has third-degree burns on 18% of total body surface area (TBSA). He is very fearful of any movement of the involved areas.

10. How is TBSA calculated in burn patients over the age of 16?
    A. Skin burn depth is calculated
    B. Rule of nines, the body is divided into areas of 9%
    C. The physician decides with the help of the burn team
    D. The physician alone decides the level of involvement

11. How do you give the client encouragement to move or participate in therapy?
    A. Provide early ADL instruction
    B. Provide adaptive equipment
    C. Provide very structured regime of exercises
    D. Allow client to direct therapy, giving him control by doing AROM

12. The posterior rotator cuff muscles include:
    A. Supraspinatus, infraspinatus, and teres minor
    B. Subscapularis, infraspinatus, and teres major
    C. Sternocleidomastoid, infraspinatus, and teres major
    D. Subscapularis, infraspinatus, and triceps

13. A chronic and recurrent experience characterized by anxiety and often expressed through defense mechanisms that impairs one's life is called:
    A. Neurosis
    B. Psychosis
    C. Mental disorder
    D. Dysphoria

14. The registration exam for the OT is administered by:
    A. AOTA
    B. NBCOT
    C. AOTF
    D. Each state's licensure board

15. Referral for occupational therapy services may come from:
    A. Physician
    B. Teacher
    C. Other therapists
    D. All of the above

16. A person with C-5 spinal cord injury would have all of the following muscle function *except*:
    A. Deltoids, shoulder flexion
    B. Biceps, elbow flexion
    C. Serratus anterior, scapular abduction
    D. Triceps, elbow extension

Use the following information to answer questions 17 through 19: Your 22-year-old male patient has Guillain-Barré syndrome. He has no speech, poor oral functioning, and all four limbs and trunk are severely involved. He has just been transferred from an acute care hospital to the rehabilitation hospital where you work.

17. Guillain-Barré syndrome is:
    A. A lower motor neuron disease
    B. A genetic disease
    C. A disease resulting from long-term abuse of alcohol
    D. A disease with total recovery

18. Symptoms of Guillain-Barré syndrome include all of the following *except*:
    A. Motor weakness and paralysis
    B. Sensory loss
    C. Compromised respiratory system
    D. Inflammation of the spinal cord

19. The *best* treatment for the first day in the rehabilitation hospital would be:
    A. Begin the evaluation but take frequent breaks
    B. Evaluate for and provide resting hand splints
    C. Set up a chin-operated communication device to call the nurse
    D. Educate the patient about occupational therapy

20. A newly admitted patient on the psychiatric unit develops a strong dislike for the OT without provocation or incident. This is an example of:
    A. Consensual validation
    B. Therapist transparency
    C. Transference
    D. Counter transference

21. Which activity is *best* for a 10-year-old boy who needs facilitation of tactile input and kinesthetic awareness?
    A. Playing a board game
    B. Rubbing different textures on his arm
    C. Playing "Simon Says"
    D. Having the child stand beside a wall and roll one way then the other

22. The executive director of AOTA is:
    A. Employed by the national association
    B. Approves policies of AOTA
    C. Elected by the ethics committee of AOTA
    D. The chairperson of the representative assembly

23. An OT receives a referral from a physician with a specific treatment recommendation. After evaluation of the patient, the OT believes a different treatment would be more effective for the patient. The *best* course of action for the OT is:
    A. Complete the different treatment, then call the physician
    B. Complete the original prescribed treatment, call the physician, and report that it is working
    C. Call the physician and suggest the OT's treatment as an alternative to the prescription
    D. Combine the two treatments and hope one is effective

Use the following information to answer questions 24 and 25: One of the greatest dangers for a person with C-4 spinal cord injury is autonomic dysreflexia. The occupational therapist must know how to recognize and manage this.

24. The symptoms of autonomic dysreflexia include all of the following *except*:
    A. Increased perspiration
    B. Flushing of the skin
    C. Dry, hot skin
    D. Severe headache

25. The *best* response if your client exhibits autonomic dysreflexia is:
    A. Keep the patient upright in the wheelchair and get immediate medical assistance
    B. Check the leg bag tubing for an obstruction, check blood pressure, and continue therapy if no problems are noted
    C. Recline the patient and get immediate medical assistance
    D. Ask someone to inform the nurse that the patient is complaining of a headache

26. All of the following are common pathological causes of feeding and swallowing disorders in the elderly *except:*
    A. Stroke
    B. Head trauma
    C. Liver or kidney disease
    D. Degenerative neurological disorders

27. The development of coma in a person with Alzheimer's disease can be the result of all of the following *except*:
    A. Myocardial infarction
    B. Overmedication
    C. Stroke
    D. Head trauma

28. Adverse drug reactions are common in the elderly. Which statement is *not* true about these reactions in older adults?
    A. Toxic reaction can occur even at low drug dosages
    B. Reactions can include drowsiness, depression, confusion, or dizziness
    C. Medications can cause involuntary movements or drug-related Parkinsonism
    D. Over-the-counter drugs such as antacids, cold medicines, and laxatives are safe

29. Alternatives to restraining elderly residents who are unsteady on their feet include all of the following *except:*
    A. Address possible low vision problems
    B. Reading material or books on tapes
    C. Soft slippers and increased ambulation
    D. Meaningful activities to participate in

30. Activities that are calming to the sensory integrative systems include all of the following *except:*
    A. Defy gravity, up and down
    B. Swinging or sustained movements
    C. Heavy touch, massage
    D. Decreased motor activities

31. All of the following techniques are effective in the behavioral management of persons with brain injury *except:*
    A. Praise efforts of the client to regain control
    B. Give an alternative such as "I'll have to report this behavior to the team"
    C. Create a plan or agreement to accomplish tasks
    D. Ignore negative, attention-seeking behaviors and comments

32. At what age is the highest frequency of epilepsy seen?
    A. Birth to 10 years
    B. 11 to 39 years
    C. 40 to 69 years
    D. 70 years plus

33. Complications of spasticity include all of the following *except:*
    A. Hypotonic muscles around joints leads to poor support
    B. Poor skin hygiene
    C. Contractures
    D. Decubiti

34. The following clinical signs are noted in your patient: ataxic gait, hypotonia, dysmetria, and dysdiadochokinesia. From these clinical signs, which part of the brain has sustained damage?
    A. Parietal lobe
    B. Premotor cortex
    C. Cerebellum
    D. Basal ganglia

35. An example of an eclectic frame of reference is:
    A. Behavior modification
    B. Object relations
    C. Cognitive behavioral
    D. Task-oriented treatment

36. What would be the *best* treatment option for a child with sensory integration, particularly vestibular problems?
    A. Reading a book in a big, overstuffed chair in the library
    B. Playing on the fixed monkey bars in the schoolyard
    C. Playing on the swing set in the schoolyard
    D. Being wrapped up tight in a blanket in a comfortably warm room

37. All of the following statements are true concerning phantom sensation following limb loss in adults *except*:
    A. Almost all adults experience phantom sensations following limb loss
    B. 60% of all patients experience phantom pain
    C. Phantom pain is considered a disturbance in body image
    D. The existence of neurological scheme ends with the actual physical loss of the limb

38. A patient with left-sided hemiplegia is asked to draw a clock. All of the following are being evaluated *except*:
    A. Visual perception
    B. Visual sequencing
    C. Visual constructive ability
    D. Ability to tell time

39. Which assessment is designed to identify developmental delays of pre-academic skills in children?
    A. Movement Assessment of Infants Screening Test
    B. Erhardt Developmental Prehension Assessment
    C. Miller Assessment for Preschoolers
    D. Peabody Developmental Motor Scales

40. What would be the *best* cognitive behavioral activity to use in occupational therapy?
    A. One that teaches ADL skills with emphasis on education and successful completion
    B. One that increases sensory input and facilitates an adaptive response
    C. One that identifies activities for fulfilling occupational roles
    D. One that emphasizes art and drawing with the meaning of symbols

41. Which of the following statements is true about spasticity?
    A. May aid in the prevention of osteoporosis
    B. May aid in the prevention of muscle atrophy
    C. May aid in the prevention of deep vein thrombosis
    D. All of the above

42. The assessment of cognition includes attention, orientation, memory, mental status, and:
    A. Executive function
    B. Motor apraxia
    C. Perceptual function
    D. Visual motor function

43. Gradation of an activity means:
    A. Assigning a grade to the patient's completed task
    B. Adjusting the pace and modifying the demand to meet the patient's maximum capabilities
    C. Assigning minimal to maximum assistance to the task depending on the amount of assistance the patient needs from the therapist
    D. Encouraging the patient to try one more time to complete an uncompleted task

44. All of the following demonstrate good listening skills *except:*
    A. Lean slightly backwards
    B. Make eye contact
    C. Body appears open
    D. Face client squarely

Use the following information to answer questions 45 through 48: You are an occupational therapist working in a specialized facility for people with head traumas. Your facility treats clients from subacute to community reentry and outpatient. The facility uses Rancho Los Amigos (RLA) levels to assign clients to different programs. You have clients in all the different programs.

45. When working with patients with head injuries, at what level does sensory stimulation treatment seem *most* appropriate?
    A. Level I
    B. Level III
    C. Level V
    D. Level VII

46. When would the same sensory stimulation treatment be the *most* inappropriate?
    A. Level I
    B. Level II
    C. Level III
    D. Level IV

47. At what level is repetition and practice of tasks *most* appropriate?
    A. Level IV
    B. Level V
    C. Level VI
    D. Level VII

48. Level VIII is purposeful and appropriate interaction with the environment. All of the following would be effective treatment for a client at level VIII *except:*
    A. Cognitive rehabilitation
    B. Vocational rehabilitation
    C. Work hardening programs
    D. Community mobility training

49. The *best* response to a person who is clearly psychotic, telling you how the FBI and CIA are chasing him, is:
    A. "I have to go now"
    B. "That's very interesting, tell me more about that"
    C. "Now think about this, you know it can't be true, it's part of your disease"
    D. "That sounds crazy to me, I can't talk to you when you say these things"

50. Which activity is *most* appropriate for a person hearing threatening voices?
    A. A 1,000-piece puzzle
    B. A tie-dyed t-shirt
    C. Leather wallet with written directions
    D. Learning a simple word processing computer program

Section Four Answers and Explanations

1. Answer: D

The infant's lower lip drops, the tongue moves forward, and the head turns when the rooting reflex is stimulated. This reflex can persist up to 7 months while the infant is asleep and is important to feeding. The grasp reflex is secondary to pressure on the palm of an infant. The galant reflex involves stroking the skin between the 12th rib and iliac crest and it persists in the newborn for 2 months. The primary righting reflex is elicited with pressure on the feet, ankles kneaded, or nape of neck tickled.

2. Answer: D

A member of good standing in AOTA has paid dues, followed the code of ethics, and met any other qualifications. A significant contribution to the field is awarded with honors but is not required to be in good standing.

3. Answer: B

Goal-directed (level 4) actions use visual cues. Basic ADLs are performed, but nonvisual safety hazards are unrecognized. Attention span is about 1 hour. Level 5 uses trial and error, can recall several steps, and can complete basic ADLs. Level 6 is the highest level and represents no disability. Level 3 can perform manual actions with tactile cues. Attention span is about 30 minutes and needs repetition of steps.

4. Answer: B

A simple, familiar task with limited steps and visual cues is best. "Simon Says" is best for level 2. Budgeting and a model airplane are best for level 5.

5. Answer: A

Although all answers have merit, patient load requirements has the greatest impact on the number of staff required. OTs who treat each patient 2 hours per day cannot treat as many patients as OTs who treat each patient for 30 minutes per day.

6. Answer: D

AOTA membership is open to OTs, OTAs, and OT students.

7. Answer: D

Performance areas in occupation of *The Practice Framework* include ADLs, IADLs, education, social participation, work, and play/leisure.

8. Answer: C

A classic sign of neglect is noted when half of the body is neglected in shaving, dressing, or washing. Motor apraxia would be a sequencing problem. Ideational apraxia would be noted if the patient were handed a shirt and the patient did not know what to do with it. Astereognosis is the inability to identify objects through touch alone.

9. Answer: C

MMT is invalid when a client does not have voluntary control of muscle function. A, B, and D would all benefit from ongoing assessment of muscle function.

10. Answer: B

The body surface is divided into areas of 9% or multiples of 9.

11. Answer: D

Allowing the patient to control the AROM helps to control the level of pain.

12. Answer: A

The rotator cuff muscles include the "SIT" muscles: supraspinatus, infraspinatus, and teres minor. Subscapularis is an anterior cuff muscle. C and D are not cuff muscles.

13. Answer: A

Neurosis appears as a symptom. Reality testing is intact. Anxiety, somatoform, dissociative sexual, and dysthymic disorders are examples. Psychosis is not reality bound. Mental disorder is distress or disability from behavioral, biological, or psychological cause. Dysphoria is an unpleasant mood.

14. Answer: B

Only NBCOT administers the OT exam.

15. Answer: D

Any person can make a referral to an occupational therapist; however, third party insurance providers often require a physician's order for reimbursement of services.

16. Answer: D

The triceps are innervated by C-7 and C-8. Deltoid, biceps, and serratus anterior are innervated at C-5 or above.

17. Answer: A

Guillain-Barré is a lower motor neuron disease. B, C, and D are not true.

18. Answer: D

Motor weakness, paralysis, sensory loss, and compromised respiratory system, to some degree, are all symptoms of Guillain-Barré. Inflammation is limited to the myelin sheath and PNS.

19. Answer: C

The best choice for the first day is setting up a device to call the nurse to improve communication and self-control of the environment.

20. Answer: C

Transference is a psychoanalytic term used to describe projected thoughts or feelings onto the therapist who represents someone from the past. Consensual validation is when group members check their perceptions with other group members. Therapist transparency is when the therapist reveals more about himself or herself to confirm or disconfirm the patient's perception. Counter transference refers to the therapist's projection onto the patient.

21. Answer: D

Although all the activities provide either some tactile input or some kinesthetic awareness, rolling on the wall provides both.

22. Answer: A

The executive director of AOTA is a full-time employee of the association. Policies of AOTA are approved by the representative assembly (RA). The ethics committee or the RA does not elect the executive director.

23. Answer: C

This situation is common in practice. The OT should call the doctor and initiate a professional conversation about the assessment and suggested treatment.

24. Answer: C

Autonomic dysreflexia includes symptoms of increased perspiration, flushing, and headache.

25. Answer: A

Autonomic dysreflexia is an immediate medical emergency. Keep the patient upright and get medical assistance immediately. Do check the leg bag tubing for obstruction but do not continue treatment.

26. Answer: C

Liver or kidney disease may affect the patient's interest in food, diet requirements, or digestion, but does not affect swallowing.

27. Answer: A

B, C, and D can cause a coma in a person with Alzheimer's disease. A head injury from a fall may appear to be a seizure. The MI is less likely to be the cause of the coma unless it resulted in anoxia.

28. Answer: D

Over-the-counter medicines can also cause adverse drug reactions, especially when mixed with prescriptions. The longer an individual is on a medication, the greater the likelihood of drug reactions. Drugs are a major cause of dizziness in persons over age 60.

29. Answer: C

Increased ambulation does improve unsteadiness but appropriate footwear that provides support must be worn. A, B, and D provide additional alternatives to restraints.

30. Answer: A

Mildred Ross describes this as an alerting activity.

31. Answer: B

This approach is evidence of a power struggle and is often perceived as threatening by the patient who can easily become defensive. A, C, and D are all behavioral techniques aimed at increasing positive reinforcement to increase desired behaviors.

32. Answer: A

Newborns to youth have the highest frequency of epilepsy. Numbers decrease in the 11 to 69 age range and then increase again at 70 due to increased health problems and medications.

33. Answer: A

Hypotonic muscles are low tone which leads to lack of support of joints. Spastic muscles are hypertonic. B, C, and D are all complications of spasticity.

34. Answer: C

The function of the cerebellum is the execution of smooth, coordinated, and properly timed movement. Ataxic gait is an uncoordinated gait. Hypotonia is a decrease in muscle tone. Dysmetria is the inability to direct movement and is characterized by reaching past objects. Dysdiadochokinesia is the inability for rapid, repeated, alternating movements. Clinical signs of parietal lobe damage include sensory disorders, apraxia, and perceptual problems. Clinical signs of premolar cortex damage include motor apraxia and difficulty with tasks that require sensory guidance. Clinical signs of basal ganglia damage include akinesia, bradykinesia, dystonia, and perseveration.

35. Answer: B

Eclecticism refers to the selection and organized blending of compatible features from a variety of sources. Object relations is a blending of humanistic-existential, Freudian, and Jungian theories. A and C are specific frames of reference that have been researched for measurable outcomes. D is not a frame of reference but refers to Fidler's group model.

36. Answer: C

Vestibular treatment with swings or suspended equipment is most effective, although the fixed monkey bars may be able to provide some movement. A and D provide no movement and therefore no treatment, however, are likely to be preferred by a child with vestibular problems.

37. Answer: D

Almost all adults experience some sensation, with over half experiencing pain. Phantom pain does disturb body image but may aid in rehabilitation in that the patient continues to have body perception during training. Phantom pain exists because the neurological scheme continues after loss of the actual limb.

38. Answer: D

The clock drawing task is a non-standardized but effective tool to evaluate perceptual problems often seen in those people with CVAs and left-sided weakness. The task is perceptual, not cognitive, and does not evaluate the ability to tell time.

39. Answer: C

The MAP is a preschool screening test designed to assess developmental delays in pre-academic skills. The MAI-ST identifies movement patterns in infants 2 to 18 months. The EDPA measures changes in hand functioning. The Peabody assesses fine and gross motor skills in children up to age 7 years.

40. Answer: A

This activity could estimate cognitive functioning and increase a person's self-knowledge. B is sensory integrative in its approach. C is part of the habituation subsystem in the model of human occupation, and D is part of object relations theory.

41. Answer: D

Although serious complications can be associated with spasticity, there are some important benefits also associated. Spasticity aids in the prevention of osteoporosis due to the pressure exerted on the bone by the muscle. Calcium loss from the bone is decreased. Muscle atrophy is prevented due to the contracted state of the muscle. Prevention of DVT is achieved by a decreased probability of blood pooling in the lower extremities when spasticity is present.

42. Answer: A

Executive function includes the ability to organize and carry out a task. This includes making decisions, sequencing, problem solving, and judgment. B, C, and D are tested in perceptual evaluations.

43. Answer: B

Gradation is adapting an activity higher or lower to provide adequate challenge but guarantee success in the patient. All other answers are false.

44. Answer: A

Good listening skills include all of the answers, except the therapist should lean slightly forward toward the client. Facing the client, maintaining eye contact, and appearing relaxed and open tells the client "I'm here for you."

45. Answer: A

Level I, no response, and level II, generalized response, are appropriate for sensory stimulation. Level III, localized response, may further benefit, but they can begin to handle other activities.

46. Answer: D

Level IV, confused agitated, is a heightened state of activity with agitation. Sensory stimulation would not be appropriate for this client as it would likely confuse the client more.

47. Answer: C

Level VI is the confused but appropriate level where clients benefit from repetition and practice in a safe environment. The levels before VI are confused, inappropriate, or agitated and tasks may not be practiced successfully. Level VII is community based, practice is in the community.

48. Answer: A

Cognitive rehabilitation is most heavy in levels V and VI with complex tasks managed at level VII. Level VIII would have mastered the skills.

49. Answer: B

Leaving or confronting a person with delusions isolates the person. Delusions are unreal beliefs that cannot be cleared with facts. Until the person's thoughts clear with medication, the best approach is to validate the person's feelings without feeding into the delusion.

50. Answer: B

A, C, and D require too much attention for this patient to successfully complete. The tie-dyed t-shirt is a success-oriented project because even if mistakes are made because the client is distracted, the shirt will usually come out well.

Section Five

1. Low back pain is a common problem for most of the adult population. The aging process results in loss of water in the disc and the joint space narrows. What role does occupational therapy play in reducing the risk of back injury?
    A. Teaching strengthening programs
    B. Redesigning work stations
    C. Observation of client body mechanics
    D. Prevention and retraining education

2. Your client experienced a myocardial infarction 3 days ago and is feeling anxious. He is medically stable and his doctor has explained what has happened, but the client remains anxious. What is the *best* approach for rehabilitation of this client?
    A. Educate the family to client's decrease in activity tolerance
    B. Teach client energy conservation and work simplification
    C. Begin graded resistive exercise program
    D. Stress reduction and long-term relaxation techniques

3. The BTE is an electromagnetic device that has 20 interchangeable tools and utilizes a computer to calibrate and calculate data in a qualitative way. For what type of program is this piece of equipment ideal?
    A. Cardiac rehabilitation
    B. CVA motor learning program
    C. Work rehabilitation
    D. Sensory integration programs

4. Play is often seen as child's work. Children who do not play are ill-prepared for adulthood. In the hospital the OT should foster play by doing all of the following *except:*
    A. Structure the activities to prevent spontaneous play
    B. Role model the excitement of exploration
    C. Alternate solitary activity with social activity
    D. Have activities to develop problem solving and decision making

5. An OT is asked to give a presentation to a local advocacy group for adults with mental health problems. The *most* effective presentation would be:
    A. Reviewing assessments such as BaFPE, ACL, KELS
    B. Discussing problems that adults with mental health diagnoses might have and how occupational therapy addresses those problems
    C. A demonstration of new computer programs to refer patients to community placements
    D. Teaching basic counseling techniques so the audience can use them with their consumers

6. What governmental program provides medical coverage for people age 65 and over?
    A. Medicaid
    B. Medicare
    C. SSI/SSD
    D. Welfare and Section 8

7. The purpose of documentation includes all of the following *except:*
    A. Data for research, education, reimbursement, treatment
    B. Serial and legal record of therapeutic intervention
    C. Facilitate communication among health care professionals
    D. Cover the therapist in case there is an ethical problem

Use the following information to answer questions 8 and 9: A 25-year-old female psychiatric patient puts on dark sunglasses every time she passes you in the hallway. During your initial assessment, you ask her about this behavior. She tells you that the glasses prevent you from putting horrible thoughts in her head.

8.   This behavior is an example of:
    A. Thought insertion
    B. Delusions of reference
    C. Hypervigilance
    D. Magical thinking

9.   The *most* appropriate response for the OT would be:
    A. "That's true"
    B. "Why would you think that?"
    C. "It is inappropriate to wear sunglasses indoors"
    D. "You must be feeling uneasy with me in this interview"

10.   A needs assessment can provide information about the need for a new occupational therapy program. All of the following are good sources of information *except:*
    A. Focus group of patients
    B. Survey to physicians
    C. Demographic information
    D. Etiology information

11.   RSD is a debilitating, progressive disease. Your client is in the first stage of RSD with classic signs of hand edema, fear of ROM, and shoulder and hand pain. What is your *first* priority in treatment?
    A. Reduction of edema
    B. AROM with emphasis on self ROM
    C. Aggressive PROM to prevent stage II progression
    D. Establish rapport with patient while talking about ADLs

12.   Occupational therapists can assess peripheral nerve function in their clients with many quick screening tests available to clinicians. The simple test for radial nerve function would be:
    A. Thumb and little finger opposition
    B. Wrist extension
    C. Gross grasp assessment with dynamometer
    D. Pinch thumb and index finger

13.   Personality factors such as rigidity, hostility, manipulation, passive-aggressive, and dependent behaviors are associated with:
    A. Arthritis
    B. Multiple sclerosis
    C. Chronic pain syndrome
    D. Any patient coping with chronic pain or chronic disabilities

14.   Swan neck deformity can result from a rupture of the lateral slips of the extensor digitorum communis (EDC) tendon. What finger position would result?
    A. MCP subluxation
    B. DIP hyperextension and PIP flexion
    C. MCP ulnarly deviated
    D. PIP hyperextension and DIP flexion

Use the following information to answer questions 15 through 18: John is a 24-year-old single male recently admitted to the inpatient psychiatric unit. He lives at home with his parents and depends on them for financial support because he spends all his money. He presents as agitated, with sporadic concentration and racing thoughts. He believes that he is a famous rock star and is shocked that you do not recognize him. He says he cannot wait to start a project in OT.

15. John's symptoms *most* closely resemble which disorder?
    A. Obsessive-compulsive disorder
    B. Generalized anxiety disorder
    C. Bipolar disorder
    D. Attention deficit hyperactivity disorder

16. John's belief that he is a rock star is an example of:
    A. A hallucination
    B. A delusion, grandiose type
    C. Paranoid ideation
    D. Malingering

17. Which of the following would be the *most* appropriate goal for this patient?
    A. Increase decision making
    B. Improve level of independence in ADLs
    C. Improve socialization
    D. Increase self-control

18. Which of the following activities would be the *most* appropriate to begin treatment?
    A. A tile box
    B. A 2,000-piece puzzle
    C. Wood carving
    D. Budgeting

19. Your client has extensive burns involving the anterior aspect of the UE, including the neck. Considering the position of comfort, what splint(s) would be indicated?
    A. Neck conformer
    B. Neck conformer, axillary
    C. Neck conformer, axillary, three-point elbow extension
    D. Neck conformer, axillary, three-point elbow extension, hand cock-up

20. The cause of incomplete flexion ROM of the MCP, PIP, and DIP while the wrist is in flexion is:
    A. Active insufficiency
    B. Passive insufficiency
    C. Decreased muscle strength
    D. Unknown

21. What activity is *best* to encourage the integration of primitive postural reflexes in a child?
    A. Have the child lie prone on a scooter board and spin
    B. Have the child walk on a balance beam
    C. Have the child pretend to be a dog, crawl around, roll over, and bark
    D. Have the child play a game of marbles

22. The NBCOT registration exam can be taken:
    A. After all classwork is finished
    B. After all fieldwork is finished
    C. After all classwork and fieldwork are finished
    D. After filing for licensure

23. What do the initials MORE stand for in OBRA regulations?
    A. Measurable, observable, reportable, exit behavior
    B. Measurable, observable, reportable, emotional
    C. Measurable, observable, realistic, explicit
    D. Measurable, observable, realistic, effective

24. When developing a new program for an already standing OT department, where would be the *first* place to start?
    A. Philosophy and mission statement
    B. Goals and objectives
    C. Patient services
    D. Necessary documentation

25. Scoliosis is defined as a:
    A. Narrowing of the lumbar spinal canal
    B. Gradual slipping of one vertebra on another
    C. Lateral curvature of the spine
    D. Chronic inflammation of the joints of the axial skeleton

26. Which sensory integration assessment requires additional training and certification to administer?
    A. Sensory Rating Scale
    B. Sensory Integration and Praxis Test
    C. Sensory Assessment
    D. Knickerbocker Sensorimotor History Questionnaire

27. People with Parkinson's disease often are given medication that is dopamine based, which improves movement; however, as dopamine increases what side effect also increases?
    A. Cog wheel movements
    B. Unsteady gait
    C. Psychotic features
    D. Confusion

28. People usually do not realize this, but most human beings hold their breath when they bend over to pick up something, tie their shoe, or garden. To which population is this particularly dangerous?
    A. Cardiac patients
    B. Patients with multiple sclerosis
    C. Patients with orthopedic conditions
    D. Arthritis patients

29. The approximate percent of individuals with epilepsy who can be successfully treated with antiepileptic medications is:
    A. 10%
    B. 50%
    C. 80%
    D. 100%

30. According to the American Spinal Injury Association, the term "central cord syndrome" indicates:

    A. Greater weakness in the upper extremity than the lower

    B. Greater ipsilateral proprioceptive/motor loss and contralateral loss of temperature/pin sensitivity

    C. Loss of motor function but proprioception is intact

    D. Injury to the lumbosacral nerve roots with lower extremity involvement

31. The use of aquatic therapy is on the rise. The basic principle of this modality is buoyancy. If your 25-year-old patient with head trauma weighs 250 lbs on land, what is his approximate weight in the water?

    A. 225 lbs

    B. 175 lbs

    C. 125 lbs

    D. 75 lbs

32. You receive a referral from a classroom teacher to test a 7-year-old girl who the teacher suspects possible perceptual problems are leading to difficulty in reading. The child has spastic cerebral palsy but has kept up with her peers until now. What is the *best* test to use?

    A. Developmental Test of Visual Perception (DTVP-2)

    B. Test of Visual Motor Skills (TVMS)

    C. Test of Visual Perceptual Skills (TVPS)

    D. Motor-Free Visual Perception Test (MVPT)

33. AOTPAC is the political action committee that represents the profession of occupational therapy. AOTPAC suggests all occupational therapists must take an active role in national legislation that affects occupational therapy. When writing a letter to your congressperson or your senator:

    A. Explain how the issue will impact you and your community

    B. Avoid form letters

    C. Be constructive in your proposals, offering professional advice

    D. All of the above

34. You are about to treat a patient bedside but "Methicillin Resistant Staphylococcus Aureus" (MRSA) is noted in his chart. What does this mean?

    A. The patient is an IV abusing or recreational drug user

    B. The patient is ventilator dependent and requires oxygen monitoring

    C. The patient has an infection that cannot be treated with traditional antibiotics

    D. The patient is HIV positive and requires the use of universal precautions

35. Which assessment is *least* appropriate for evaluating independent living skills?

    A. Assessment of Motor and Process Skills (AMPS)

    B. Bay Area Functional Performance Evaluation (BaFPE)

    C. Older Americans Resources and Services Instrument (OARS)

    D. Fugl-Meyer Scale (FM)

36. What is the *first* thing a therapist should do when washing his or her hands?

    A. Turn on the water and adjust the temperature

    B. Apply soap to hands

    C. Remove rings and put them on the sink's edge

    D. Pull out a length of paper towel

37. If assessment on the Baltimore Therapeutic Equipment (BTE) simulator suggests that the maximum a female worker's compensation client can lift at this time is 7 lbs, which item in her home will she be unable to lift?

    A. A jumbo box of cereal

    B. A gallon of milk

    C. A blow dryer

    D. A portable telephone

38. Understanding an individual's weight bearing precautions is essential to addressing mobility with a client. Which level allows a small amount of weight to be applied by the affected leg?

    A. Toe touch weight bearing (TTWB)

    B. Partial weight bearing (PWB)

    C. Weight bearing as tolerated (WBAT)

    D. Full weight bearing (FWB)

39. Rotter introduced a concept that describes one's belief in personal responsibility for an outcome of an action. When a person believes that he or she is personally responsible for life events rather than life events being controlled by outside influences, this is called:

    A. Competence

    B. Locus of control

    C. Internal locus of control

    D. External locus of control

40. The term that defines the level of proficiency in a specific activity or task is known as:

    A. Skill

    B. Ability

    C. Autonomy

    D. Order

41. Which of the following outcomes or goals is applicable to Claudia Allen's cognitive disabilities frame of reference?

    A. To achieve competence in social roles

    B. To achieve mastery of developmental milestones

    C. To increase organization, function, and adaptation in occupational performance

    D. To improve thinking and performance in various activities with a just right challenge

Use the following information to answer questions 42 through 44: Your client is a 64-year-old woman with rheumatoid joint disease. She is currently being seen three times a week in an outpatient program. The client exhibits multiple joint involvement in the wrist and hands. Currently in the clinic, the client is using paraffin, exercises, and experimenting with adaptive equipment. In addition, the client is participating in her home program. Presently, the client is on NSAIDs and a DMARD (disease-modifying anti-rheumatic drug).

42. NSAIDs are:

    A. Nonsteroidal anti-inflammatory drugs

    B. Expensive medication

    C. New steroid anti-inflammatory drugs

    D. Other disease-modifying drug

43. The client is reporting good results from her medication with decreased pain and stiffness, however, she is reporting a skin rash on her arms and legs. The *best* course of action is to:

    A. Question the client's response to the paraffin and discontinue use

    B. Question if the client is experiencing a side effect of the disease-modifying drug

    C. Question the client about past allergic reactions to aspirin or NSAIDs

    D. Consult with a family member regarding possible exposure to home contaminants

44. What is the *first* priority in choosing a piece of adaptive equipment for this particular client?
    A. A long-handled reacher so she does not have to reach so far
    B. A long-handled bath sponge to make showering easier
    C. A bar stool in the kitchen so she can rest during homemaking chores
    D. A piece of equipment that the client wants to use

45. Parkinson's disease is a movement disorder characterized by all of the following symptoms *except:*
    A. Postural instability
    B. Bradykinesia
    C. Rigidity
    D. Intentional tremor

46. What is the lowest level of OT that can provide supervision of OT aides, technicians, care extenders, all levels of OTAs, volunteers, and level I fieldwork students?
    A. Entry-level OTs with less than 1 year experience
    B. Intermediate-level OTs
    C. Advance-level OTs with 5 or more years' experience
    D. Any physical therapist

47. An entry-level OTA with less than 1 year of experience must have close supervision by an OT or intermediate/advanced OTA. How is close supervision defined?
    A. Constant, direct supervision of all treatment sessions
    B. Daily, direct contact at the work site
    C. Direct contact at least every 2 weeks with telephone contact more often
    D. Direct contact once a month with telephone contact as needed

48. An OT works in a school system with children who have deficits in sensory integration. The OT is utilizing A. J. Ayers' frame of reference to improve sensory integrative function and performance. How will this goal be *best* achieved?
    A. By controlling sensory input to elicit an adaptive response
    B. Through movement patterns requiring new responses
    C. Through direct involvement in activities that will develop work skills later in life
    D. Through stimulating task and interpersonal skill development

49. According to the World Health Organization International Classification, what is the correct definition of disability?
    A. Abnormality or loss pertaining to either psychological or physical origin
    B. Restriction to perform an activity within a normal range of functioning
    C. A disadvantage that limits or prevents fulfillment of normal role performance
    D. Disruption in the roles of daily living

50. The AOTA position paper on the use of physical agent modalities (PAMs) would allow the use of paraffin in all of the following cases *except:*
    A. As a warm-up for exercise for a client with a hand trauma
    B. Combined with other PAMs as a pain reliever
    C. Before doing keyboarding with a client with arthritis
    D. While trying to increase ROM in an elbow with chronic pain

Section Five Answers and Explanations

1. Answer: D
Industrial prevention programs and education in chronic pain programs are essential roles in occupational therapy. A, B, and C are components of prevention and retraining education.

2. Answer: D
Anxiety must be dealt with first to address immediate physical limitations and long-term lifestyle changes. A, B, and C are important treatment components but are secondary to reducing anxiety.

3. Answer: C
The BTE is commonly used for evaluation and treatment in a work rehabilitation program. Although the BTE might be used for cardiac rehabilitation, it is unlikely to be used for motor learning after a CVA or for sensory integration programs.

4. Answer: A
Spontaneous play is an essential component of a child's work.

5. Answer: B
The OT must keep in mind the target audience when developing presentations. This audience would benefit from learning about the problems adults with mental illness face and how occupational therapy can address the weaknesses.

6. Answer: B
Medicare is for those age 65 and over. Medicaid is a state health program for the poor. SSI/SSD is income for people over age 65 or people with disabilities. Welfare and Section 8 are state income programs for the poor.

7. Answer: D
Although documentation can help a health care professional in case there is an ethical claim, the purpose of documentation is to protect the consumer. Research, communication, and serial records are all benefits of proper documentation.

8. Answer: A
Thought insertion is a delusion in which the patient believes that thoughts are being implanted by an outside force. Delusions of reference is the belief that behavior of others refers to oneself. Hypervigilance is continuous scanning of the environment for self-protection. Magical thinking is believing one has magical powers to cause something to happen.

9. Answer: D
The occupational therapist should consider using empathy to minimize tensions because the patient is delusional. This response, unlike the others, will convey understanding and assist in establishing rapport. A, B, and C will likely increase the patient's defenses.

10. Answer: D
Focus groups, surveys, demographics, questionnaires, key informants, and literature reviews are all excellent sources of data for a needs assessment. Etiology information is not helpful unless it directly relates to a high environmental incidence in your area. Needs assessments focus on the need for services, not the cause of diseases.

11. Answer: A
All of the answers are important to the treatment of RSD; however, edema should be the therapist's first concern.

12. Answer: B
The wrist extensors are innervated by the radial nerve. Thumb and little finger opposition can be a median nerve test. Gross grasp is not a specific test. Pinching the thumb and index finger can be an ulnar nerve test. More detailed evaluation is needed to specifically identify median/ulnar problems.

13. Answer: D

Dependency needs in the early phase of adjustment to a chronic disease can be seen in chronic pain, multiple sclerosis, arthritis, and other long-term diseases.

14. Answer: D

Swan neck can be caused by other factors, but the classic position is PIP hyperextension and DIP flexion. MCP subluxation is articular instability secondary to capsular weakness and muscle imbalance. DIP hyperextension and PIP flexion is boutonniere deformity. MCP ulnarly deviated is generally associated with weak collateral ligaments.

15. Answer: C

The symptoms most closely resemble a manic episode of bipolar disorder.

16. Answer: B

The patient genuinely believes that he is a famous person who has achieved great accomplishment. An unreal belief is a delusion. Hallucinations are perceptual, not cognitive. There is no suggestion of paranoid thinking. Malingering is an intentional act to deceive and is not considered a mental disorder.

17. Answer: D

The patient must be able to modify his own behavior to the environment to accomplish the other goals mentioned. A, B, and C are relevant after poor self-control is stabilized first.

18. Answer: A

A tile box project would provide structure and repetition to sustain attention and attain mastery. The puzzle and budgeting are too lengthy and unstructured for the initial treatment sessions. Wood carving should be avoided due to the sharp utensils until the patient is stabilized.

19. Answer: D

One splint alone will not be sufficient; all are required.

20. Answer: B

Due to the stretch of the extensors over more than one joint, the length of the muscle would not allow full flexion to occur.

21. Answer: C

Playing dog involves extended arms and head movement. Spinning on a scooter board is a vestibular activity. The balance beam activity may be too advanced for this child. Marbles are a fine motor activity.

22. Answer: C

The NBCOT exam can be taken only after all classwork and fieldwork are completed. State licensure requires applicants to have completed the NBCOT process.

23. Answer: C

Measurable, observable, realistic, explicit.

24. Answer: A

The philosophy and mission statement are the foundation for the existing programs as well as the new program. Goals, objectives, patient services, and documentation are developed only after the philosophy and mission statement are reviewed.

25. Answer: C

Scoliosis is often noted in young females. Routine testing in schools throughout the country screens for this lateral curvature of the spine.

26. Answer: B

The SIPT requires pediatric experience, specific training, and knowledge of statistics and measurement. Three courses are offered by Sensory Integration International. The Sensory Rating Scale is for ages 0 to 3 years and takes 20 minutes to give. The Sensory Assessment is for ages 5 to 18 years and is standardized. The KSHQ is a questionnaire given to parents about their child's behavior.

27. Answer: C

This side effect makes sense if you think about the two diseases: Parkinson's and schizophrenia. People with Parkinson's have a decreased level of dopamine and people with schizophrenia have too much dopamine. As the medication increases to improve movement, psychotic features may present.

28. Answer: A

Bending over is a concern for all the diagnoses listed, but holding their breath while bending over is of particular danger for cardiac patients as the two combined adds additional stress on the heart.

29. Answer: C

According to data collected in 1996, 80% of all people with epilepsy can be successfully treated. Although the disease is not cured, medication can reduce seizure activity modifying the disease process to reduce further damage to the CNS.

30. Answer: A

Central cord syndrome occurring in the cervical region results in sacral sensory sparing and greater weakness in the UE than the LE. B is Brown-Sequard syndrome. C is anterior cord syndrome. D is cauda equina syndrome.

31. Answer: C

The biomechanical factor shows that approximately 50% of the body weight is supported by the concept of buoyancy.

32. Answer: D

The MVPT provides a quick assessment of visual perceptual abilities without requiring the child to have motor skills. Since the child has cerebral palsy, motor skills may be a problem. Her age of 7 is within the age range of all the assessments.

33. Answer: D

When writing legislative letters, include all of the items, as well as address the letter correctly, keep comments to the point, and be respectful.

34. Answer: C

All of the items are false except C. It is important that the occupational therapist be aware of MRSA because the therapist is at risk of becoming infected or passing the infection on to others. Follow hospital guidelines for gowning, wearing gloves, and wearing eye protection.

35. Answer: D

The Fugl-Meyer Scale is a measure of motor recovery after stroke. All the other assessments include independent living skills subtests.

36. Answer: D

Pull out a paper towel so that it will be ready to dry your clean hands without touching the dispenser. Turn on the water and wet hands before adding soap. Rub hand and wrists vigorously for at least 15 seconds. Wash around rings, do not remove. Rinse well and dry hands. Use paper towel to turn off water. Do not touch the wastebasket.

37. Answer: B

A gallon of milk weighs over 8 lbs (128 oz/16 oz per pound = 8 lbs plus the container weight). All the other items weigh about 2 lbs.

38. Answer: B

TTWB does not allow any weight but allows the toe to be used for balance. WBAT allows weight to be applied until pain. FWB has no restrictions.

39. Answer: C

Rotter called this general concept locus of control. Internal locus of control is when a person feels personally responsible for life events rather than life events being controlled by outside influences. External locus of control refers to a belief that outside forces are causing events to happen. Competence is efficacy in meeting environmental demands.

40. Answer: A

Ability is a general trait referring to genetic influences and learning during one's life. Autonomy is shown by one's ability to make choices and have control over one's environment. Order refers to a desired, symptom-free state of being.

41. Answer: D

Allen's theory is suited for persons with physical and cognitive deficits who can benefit by learning how to compensate for his or her decreased abilities. A refers to Mosey's frame of role acquisition. B refers to a developmental frame such as Llorens'. C refers to the model of human occupation.

42. Answer: A

Common NSAIDs are inexpensive over-the-counter medications such as aspirin or ibuprofen. These are considered the frontline approach to the management of arthritis. NSAIDs are not disease modifying but do treat the symptoms.

43. Answer: B

The client is on a DMARD such as oral gold compound (Ridaura/auranofin), which attempts to halt the progression of arthritic changes. Gold has many side effects, including skin rash, diarrhea, and irritation of the oral mucosa.

44. Answer: D

The client may have difficulty holding on to any long-handled piece of equipment. The bar stool may be a good idea, but since the client is living in her own home and has no cognitive problems, the best approach is for her to try out different pieces of equipment and then choose what she thinks will be most helpful.

45. Answer: D

Intentional tremor is a tremor on movement, usually seen in multiple sclerosis. The tremor associated with Parkinson's disease is a resting tremor or pill rolling movement. A, B, and C are characteristics of the disease.

46. Answer: A

A new OT can supervise all levels of OT personnel except a level II fieldwork student. The new graduate's supervision is not required but highly recommended.

47. Answer: B

A new graduate OTA must be supervised at the site with daily direct contact. Intermediate or advanced OTAs can have routine or general supervision.

48. Answer: A

Ayers believed that adaptive responses could be achieved when sensation is organized and situations provide a "just right" challenge with built-in success. B refers to Gilfoyle and Grady's frame of spatiotemporal adaptation, which emphasizes the role of movement in one's environment. C refers to Reilly's occupational behavior, which emphasizes humans' innate need to master their environment through play and work. D refers to Mosey's role acquisition, in which humans' desire for mastery leads to successful adaptation in a variety of roles, including ADLs, work, and play.

49. Answer: B

A defines impairment, C defines handicap, and D defines occupational performance dysfunction.

50. Answer: B

PAMs can be used by OT personnel when used in conjunction with or in preparation of purposeful activity. Simply using PAMs to reduce pain without OT treatment would not be part of occupational therapy.

Section Six

1. What is the *best* approach to prevent hypertrophic scarring of a patient with burns?

    A. The physical and occupational therapists would both range the patient daily

    B. The occupational therapist would splint the involved areas and measure the patient for pressure garments to be worn 23 hours per day

    C. Nursing would position the patient when not in therapy to prevent deformity

    D. The family would be involved to encourage the patient to comply with the rehabilitation program

2. Motor apraxia would be the *most* likely deficit when the patient:

    A. Attempts to grasp a washcloth and is unable to plan and sequence the hand movements

    B. Does not discern the foreground from the background and cannot find the soap or washcloth

    C. Becomes frustrated when having trouble with the task

    D. Did not comprehend the verbal instructions

3. Flaccidity or hypotonicity following a cerebral or spinal insult will include all of the following *except:*

    A. Decreased muscle tone

    B. Weak co-contractions

    C. Hyperactive tendon reflexes

    D. Decreased ability to resist gravity

4. A client with traumatic brain injury is in an outpatient program with the long-term goal of returning to work as an auto mechanic installing mufflers. Motorically the client is exhibiting good overall strength and coordination. In groups, he is unable to work with others or to control inappropriate behaviors. His occupational therapy program should include:

    A. Work program that includes muffler installations

    B. Pre-work hardening with emphasis on social skills for work readiness

    C. Continued work on impulse control in an inpatient hospital setting

    D. Patient is appropriate for any work program at this time

5. Group members develop standards of participation for members and expectations for leaders. What is this called?

    A. Group norms

    B. Group roles

    C. Subgrouping

    D. Task roles

6. Vestibular stimulation when used to treat a child with autism is *least* effective for improving which of the following?

    A. Communication

    B. Hyporesponsiveness

    C. Self-care

    D. Muscle tone

7. When evaluating your client's ROM, you first ask her to move the part through available AROM. What do you learn about the client through your observation?

    A. The end feel of the joint

    B. That muscle strength is good because she achieved full AROM

    C. That muscle strength is fair or above if she achieved full AROM

    D. The joint passive or accessory play

8. The relationship between the vestibular system and the cerebellum has resulted in therapy concepts that suggest slow rocking and slow or sustained inversion will result in:
    A. Reduced hypotonicity
    B. Increased hypertonicity
    C. Reduced hypertonicity
    D. Increased hypotonicity

9. Diarthrodial or synovial joints include all of the following *except:*
    A. Ball and socket
    B. Hinge
    C. Saddle
    D. Suture

10. A contraction that occurs with muscle lengthening is known as:
    A. Concentric
    B. Isometric
    C. Eccentric
    D. Isotonic

11. Which of the following does *not* describe an example of social reinforcement?
    A. Making eye contact
    B. Smiling
    C. Therapeutic self-disclosure
    D. Nodding

12. Your 5-year-old patient is coming to OT to inhibit tonic neck reflex and to increase vestibular stimulation. You ask the child to roll in a carpeted barrel or innertube with handles. What precaution is *most* important?
    A. Be aware that others watching will think the activity is unsafe
    B. Be aware that children may think of the barrel as a weapon
    C. Be aware of too much pressure on the child's hips and legs
    D. Be aware of too much vestibular input and the emotional responses

13. Which statement defines "process" in groups?
    A. Therapeutic dynamics
    B. Understanding the nature of interpersonal relationships
    C. Explicit words spoken by the members
    D. Therapeutic interventions

14. What do the initials POMR stand for?
    A. Problem-oriented medical record
    B. Performance-oriented medical record
    C. Problem-observation medical record
    D. Patient-oriented medical record

15. A client who has severe rheumatoid arthritis, but is currently in remission, wants to engage in a strengthening program. What type of exercises would be *most* beneficial?
    A. Concentric
    B. Eccentric
    C. Isotonic
    D. Isometric

16. During supination, what is moving?
    A. Ulna
    B. Radius
    C. Both ulna and radius
    D. Only the distal ulna

17. DRGs often influence hospital stay. What do the initials stand for?
    A. Diagnosis rate guide
    B. Determined and related groups
    C. Doctor's rate guide
    D. Diagnosis related groups

18. Your client has an above elbow amputation. He is fearful and hesitant to don his prosthetic device. What approach would be *most* helpful to the client?
    A. Wait until the client is ready to learn
    B. Work on a strengthening program instead
    C. Repetitive donning and removal of the prosthesis
    D. Work on stump care

19. A patient with recent hip replacement must avoid all of the following *except:*
    A. Bending while sitting
    B. Walking outside
    C. Crossed legs
    D. Crossed ankles

20. According to Anne Mosey, there are five types of nonfamilial groups simulating normal development. These groups can be organized in specific sequence to resemble the development of group interaction skills. Which of the following is *not* the correct name?
    A. Parallel
    B. Cooperative
    C. Project
    D. Egocentric

21. Occupational therapists can refer patients to:
    A. Physical therapists only in their facility
    B. Any health care professional as appropriate
    C. Only another OT
    D. Only back to the doctor from whom the patient originally came

22. Hypertension is easily detected by:
    A. Shortness of breath
    B. Headache
    C. Monitoring blood pressure with a sphygmomanometer
    D. Dizziness

23. Poor splint construction can lead to impaired function. The *most* important factor in custom splint construction is:
    A. Cosmetics—if it looks bad the client will have poor compliance
    B. During the molding, pay special attention to maintaining the arches
    C. Price—if it is too expensive the client will have poor compliance
    D. The materials used as straps

24. According to the model of human occupation frame of reference, what subsystem includes values and interests as components?
    A. Volitional
    B. Habituation
    C. Performance
    D. Environment

25. The *most* appropriate and inclusive evaluation to use with a patient suspected to have delirium would be:
    A. Allen's Cognitive Level (ACL)
    B. Bay Area Functional Performance Evaluation (BaFPE)
    C. Kohlman Evaluation of Living Skills (KELS)
    D. Mini-Mental Status Exam

26. The AOTA position paper on physical agent modalities (PAMs) states that OT personnel are allowed to use PAMs when adjunctive to or in preparation of purposeful activity *except*:
    A. When in entry-level practice
    B. When a physical therapist is available to do them
    C. When reimbursement does not pay for the service
    D. When the provider is an OTA

27. The pharmacological management of Parkinson's disease is associated with one main medication:
    A. Diazepam (Valium)
    B. L-dopa (Levodopa)
    C. NSAIDs
    D. Heparin

28. A 30-year-old female waitress worked very long hours. One evening she fell asleep resting on her right forearm. She awoke 5 hours later with signs of radial nerve injury, including wrist drop. Which splint is the *best* option for treatment?
    A. Resting hand splint
    B. Dynamic extension splint
    C. Radial gutter splint
    D. Ulnar gutter splint

29. What is the area in front of the eyes in which an object can be seen without moving the eyes?
    A. Cornea
    B. Retina
    C. Visual acuity
    D. Visual field

30. An OT has just received a referral from a physician within an acute care hospital. What is the *first* step the OT should take in problem solving the treatment process?

 A. Determine the patient's needs

 B. Write the treatment plan

 C. Assess the patient's strengths and weaknesses

 D. Plan possible intervention strategies

31. In a feeding program, puréed foods may be difficult for some clients to swallow for all of the following reasons *except:*

 A. Spicy or intense taste

 B. Unappealing appearance

 C. Lack of temperature and texture

 D. Minimal pressure requirements to chew

32. When a person with Alzheimer's cannot handle his finances but is still able to handle a demanding work schedule, what differential diagnosis might be present?

 A. Other forms of dementia in addition to Alzheimer's

 B. Pseudo-dementia due to depression

 C. CVA

 D. Anoxia from COPD

33. What over-the-counter medications are contraindicated for a person in cardiac rehabilitation?

 A. Vitamins

 B. Aspirin

 C. Tylenol brand pain relievers

 D. Alka Seltzer brand stomach and cold remedies

34. What developmental stage is marked by the drive for independence, building social relationships, defining occupational/social roles, development of intellectual skills, and values/ethics?

 A. Childhood

 B. Adolescence

 C. Young adulthood

 D. Middle adulthood

35. A patient in occupational therapy continues to deny the seriousness of his diabetes. This typical use of denial by physically ill people may be called what type of coping strategy?

 A. Cognitive strategy

 B. Behavioral strategy

 C. Avoidant strategy

 D. Problem-focused coping

36. Higher level cognitive skills, localized in the frontal lobes, are also called executive functions. All of the following are executive functions *except*:

 A. Initiation of action in new situations

 B. Ability to recognize and correct one's behavior

 C. Evaluation of one's ability with an expected performance standard

 D. Verbal discussion of behavior

Use the following information to answer questions 37 through 39: Your patient is a 70-year-old woman with a long history of congestive heart failure caused by myocarditis. She has been successfully treated with digitalis glycosides for several years. Some swelling is noted in her ankles and feet. Her endurance is slightly limited. She recently developed some weakness and incoordination in her right side.

37. Her diagnosis is likely:
    A. Myocardial infarction
    B. Pulmonary edema
    C. CVA
    D. Additional congestive heart failure

38. The client was not hospitalized but will receive therapy at home. The OT priority would be:
    A. Increase strength and ROM in right UE
    B. Increase ADL status, especially dressing
    C. Client-centered therapy
    D. Home management

39. After 2 weeks of home therapy, you notice the client is confused and lethargic, although there are no changes in her current motoric status. The *best* therapeutic response is:
    A. Continue to monitor the client's motoric status
    B. Consult with the family
    C. Consult with your OT supervisor
    D. Consult with the client's physician

40. Which law specifically prohibits discrimination based solely on an individual's disability in any program receiving federal monies?
    A. Rehabilitation Act of 1973, Section 504
    B. Education of the Handicapped Act
    C. Americans with Disabilities Act
    D. PL 94-103

41. Vertical righting reactions in children:
    A. Activate muscles to move the midline of the body into alignment with the center of gravity
    B. Activate muscles to lift the head to either side
    C. Are present at birth
    D. All of the above

42. When a child is supported in the supine position and his head is gently dropped, what reflex elicits abduction and extension of the arms followed by the arms coming together in an arc?
    A. Flexor withdrawal
    B. Crossed extension
    C. Moro's
    D. Bauer's

43. Enabling a person to interact with the environment effectively and develop an accurate map of self requires all of the following systems *except*:
    A. Olfactory
    B. Somatosensory
    C. Proprioceptive
    D. Vestibular

44. All of the following are true of psychoanalytic theory and its relationship to Fidler's task group *except:*
    A. Intrapsychic conflicts are explored
    B. Emphasis is placed on the success of the end product
    C. Unmasking the unconscious is encouraged through the activity process
    D. Freud is the father of psychoanalysis

45. For a college or university to offer an entry-level degree in occupational therapy, the program must meet:
    A. Standards and guidelines for an accredited educational program for the occupational therapist
    B. Core values and attitudes of occupational therapy practice
    C. Standards of practice for occupational therapy
    D. Occupational therapy code of ethics

46. A patient who believes he cannot meet the therapist's expectations in skill performance and who fears criticism is *most* likely to refuse to attend which type of occupational therapy group?
    A. Weekend planning group (leisure)
    B. Community trip to the mall (socialization)
    C. Current events group (psychoeducational)
    D. Arts and crafts (task)

47. AOTA defines occupational therapy practitioners as:
    A. An OT
    B. An OT and OTA
    C. An OT, OTA, or OT aide
    D. Any person who practices occupational therapy

48. The *Occupational Therapy Roles* paper is an official document of the AOTA. What roles are defined in this document?
    A. OT and OTA practitioners
    B. Clinical and education fieldwork educators
    C. Supervisor, administrator, consultant, and entrepreneur
    D. All of the above

49. An occupational therapy group that has as its goal to increase the patient's planning and participation in self-care, work, and leisure is called:
    A. Coping skills
    B. Self-expression
    C. Time management
    D. Value clarification

50. A client diagnosed with narcissistic personality disorder has made a personal, sexual comment about you during occupational therapy group. What counseling strategy should you use?
    A. Self-disclosure to let the client know how offended you are by the comment
    B. Empathy to be considerate and convey understanding of the client's perspective
    C. Termination to expect the client to automatically leave your group
    D. Immediacy to discuss the therapeutic relationship and the impact on the both of you

Section Six Answers and Explanations

1. Answer: B

Pressure garments and splinting are an integral part of the program to prevent scarring. PT and OT would work together to range the involved areas; however, only pressure garments prevent scarring. Nursing and family also play an important role.

2. Answer: A

Poor motor planning and sequencing problems indicate motor apraxia. Finding the soap is an example of a figure ground problem. Frustration could be a sign of many different problems. Understanding the directions is a receptive aphasia problem.

3. Answer: C

Decreased muscle tone, weak co-contraction, and decreased ability to resist gravity are all signs of hypotonicity. Hyperactive tendon reflexes are noted in spastic hypertonicity, the opposite condition.

4. Answer: B

Clients with head injuries often require a structured pre-work hardening program that emphasizes work and social skills. At this time the client is ready for treatment but not ready for a work hardening program. The client does need to work in a group to develop skills, however, does not need inpatient hospital services. An inpatient program requires continuing medical instability.

5. Answer: A

Group norms are also known as rules of conduct. Group roles refer to the part one plays in a group. Subgrouping refers to speaking with certain members and excluding others. Task roles refer to the roles taken by members to address tasks at hand.

6. Answer: C

Vestibular stimulation has been correlated with increased verbalization, responsiveness, and muscle tone. Self-care may benefit if the child is directed to perform self-care activities. Behavioral modification techniques are helpful to address ADLs.

7. Answer: C

Informal evaluation of a client's AROM does provide the OT with initial information regarding muscle strength. The client must have a fair grade in order to achieve AROM against gravity. The therapist must provide resistance to assess a good grade, palpate to assess the end feel, or use PROM to establish joint play.

8. Answer: C

Slow rocking will result in dampening the vestibuloproprioceptors and decreasing tone throughout the body. Slow rolling and a quiet environment will also decrease tone.

9. Answer: D

The suture joint is a fibrous joint, such as a skull suture. Hinge, saddle, and ball and socket all have characteristics of diarthrodial or synovial joints, such as synovium, joint space, synovial fluid, or capsules.

10. Answer: C

Concentric is muscle shortening, isometric is no change in muscle length, and isotonic is muscle shortening.

11. Answer: C

Making eye contact, smiling, and nodding are all social reinforcers. Therapeutic self-disclosure is a skill an occupational therapist uses to support the client gaining a new awareness about himself or herself.

12. Answer: D

Too much vestibular input can cause emotional responses.

13. Answer: B
Process is the act of recognizing, examining, and understanding the nature of interpersonal relationships. Therapeutic dynamics refer to the forces within a group. Explicit words refer to the content. Therapeutic interventions refer to the technique.

14. Answer: A
The problem-oriented medical record is a type of documentation system.

15. Answer: D
Isometric exercises will reduce stress on the joint structure while exercising the soft tissue.

16. Answer: B
During supination, the proximal end of the radius spins within the radial notch. The distal end slides over the ulnar head.

17. Answer: D
Diagnosis related groups are categories that suggest the acceptable length of stay in the hospital for each diagnosis.

18. Answer: C
Repetition will help the client learn parts of the prosthetic device, enhance body scheme adjustment, allow gradation, allow for decrease of therapist cues, and will allow the client to desensitize himself to the emotional aspects of amputation. Strengthening and stump care are important but only after adjustment issues have been addressed.

19. Answer: B
Bending while sitting and crossing legs or ankles can all lead to dislocating the hip joint. Walking is safe and healthy as long as the weather is good.

20. Answer: D
Egocentric-cooperative is the correct term. At this stage, members select and implement a long-term task. At the parallel level, individuals will work side by side. At the cooperative level, the therapist is an advisor. Members can satisfy each other's social and emotional needs. Project level groups emphasize a task accomplishment with some interaction. Group development moves from parallel, project, egocentric-cooperative, cooperative, and finally to mature.

21. Answer: B
Occupational therapists can refer patients to any appropriate health care professional.

22. Answer: C
There are no clear clinical signs to detect hypertension predictably. Blood pressure must be monitored. Many people exhibit shortness of breath (SOB) for a variety of reasons. SOB may not be an indicator of high blood pressure. Headaches can occur with hypertension but also for many other reasons. Dizziness can occur with both hypertension and hypotension, as well as for other reasons.

23. Answer: B
If the arches of the hand are not maintained, deformity of the hand could result. Fit is enhanced with proper strap placement to avoid skin breakdown from rubbing.

24. Answer: A
The volitional system serves at the top of the hierarchy and energizes other subsystems to achieve goals. The three components include personal causation, values, and interests. Habituation components include roles and habits. Organization of daily activities is the main function. Performance includes skills needed to perform purposeful activities: perceptual motor, process, communication, and interactive skills. Environment is not a subsystem.

25. Answer: D

The Mini-Mental Status Exam is an excellent screening tool to track a patient's cognitive state over time. Although a formal evaluation of cognitive impairment may be done as a psychological test, the Mini-Mental Status Exam includes areas of orientation, registration, calculation, recall, language, and construction. The ACL is a cognitive test but does not address the above areas. The BaFPE includes cognitive, affective, and psychomotor. The KELS is best suited for readiness for discharge in the ADL area.

26. Answer: A

PAMs are not considered part of entry-level practice but require specialized learning. An OT can delegate the use of PAMs to an OTA with training, but as with all media, shall comply with all supervision requirements to ensure competency. OT personnel can use PAMs even if physical therapists are available or when reimbursement is not available as long as the personnel comply with state licensure laws.

27. Answer: B

The administration of Levodopa often dramatically improves symptoms, especially rigidity and bradykinesia. It remains the most common drug for the treatment of Parkinson's disease. Valium is an anti-anxiety medication. NSAIDs are anti-inflammatory and heparin is an anti-coagulant.

28. Answer: B

Although A, C, and D might provide support, the dynamic extension splint provides the best treatment for wrist drop.

29. Answer: D

A full visual field is represented by 180 degrees of vision without moving the eyes. A and B are structures in the eye. Visual acuity is the sharpness of vision.

30. Answer: C

The first step is to attain strengths and weaknesses in an initial screening and assessment followed by answer A. D is part of treatment planning.

31. Answer: A

Puréed food has a bland taste, which, added to all the other factors, may make it difficult to swallow. B, C, and D are all true.

32. Answer: B

Depression is likely the cause. All the other diagnoses would have additional signs.

33. Answer: D

Not to be used due to high sodium. The therapist should watch for signs of edema or congestive heart failure if the patient states he or she has been taking this medication and should inform the client to stop taking the medicine until consulting with the physician.

34. Answer: B

Childhood includes 6 to 12 years, young adulthood is 20 to 35 years, and middle adulthood is 35 to 50 years.

35. Answer: C

In avoidant coping, attention is focused away from the stressful source. Cognitive strategies include reasoning, appraising, and reflection. Behavioral strategies include taking action to the source of the stress. Problem-focused coping includes doing something constructive to work out the problem.

36. Answer: D

Persons with impairments in executive functioning can verbally discuss their behavior but have difficulty doing or initiating action.

37. Answer: C
The right-sided weakness indicates CVA.

38. Answer: C
A, B, and D are valuable but the client leads the therapy, especially in home care.

39. Answer: D
This client did not have another stroke, as evidenced by no decrease in motoric abilities. She likely had digitalis toxicity. The client's decrease in mobility after the stroke influenced her metabolism and excretion of the digitalis, so the same dose that was effective before the stroke is now toxic.

40. Answer: A
All the acts have influences on the education of children in the United States.

41. Answer: A
Vertical righting reactions include body righting. They are not present at birth but develop with interaction with the environment. Turning the head is part of rotational righting reactions.

42. Answer: C
Flexor withdrawal, crossed extension, and Bauer's are tested with touch pressure to the foot.

43. Answer: A
The olfactory system is a primitive, chemically based sensory system that signals the CNS about smells.

44. Answer: B
Emphasis is placed on the process of the group, not the actual end product. All other statements reflect Fidler's task group model researched at the New York Psychiatric Institute in 1965.

45. Answer: A
The other three official AOTA papers are important policies that influence education and practice of occupational therapy.

46. Answer: D
Fidler observed in her research at the New York Psychiatric Institute how patients with schizophrenia felt threatened by the act of "doing." This doing in a task group actually demonstrated their skills and functioning level. A, B, and C are not performance based.

47. Answer: B
OT practitioners are only OTs and OTAs who are certified to practice. OT aides or technicians require intense, close supervision by the OT and/or OTA.

48. Answer: D
In addition, the paper also describes the roles of faculty, program director, researcher, and scholar.

49. Answer: C
Coping skills are defined as identifying and managing stress. Self-expression is the use of various styles and skills to express thoughts, feelings, and needs. Values are identified ideas and beliefs considered personally important.

50. Answer: D
Immediacy is effectively used to discuss issues that develop between the client and the occupational therapist. An important part of immediacy is inviting the client to examine the relationship.

Section Seven

1. Which of the following is *not* true about delirium and dementia?

    A. Both include cognitive impairment

    B. Incoherent speech may result

    C. Clouding of consciousness occurs

    D. Insight may be impaired

2. Your patient is about to be discharged home within a few days. He has described a long history of dependency on alcohol and cocaine for pleasure. It is apparent to you that his family and friends also have similar patterns of abuse. What would be the *best* treatment goal considering this environment?

    A. Increase problem solving

    B. Leisure planning

    C. Increase grooming/hygiene

    D. Identify values

3. What event marks the end of the infancy stage of development?

    A. Talking

    B. Creeping

    C. Climbing stairs

    D. Bowel control

4. The *most* important role of AOTF is:

    A. Developing scholarships for OT students

    B. Facilitating a foundation and developing research in occupational therapy

    C. Fundraising for its own budget

    D. Housing the occupational therapy library

5. ROM is measured by placing the goniometer over the axis of the movement of the joint. When measuring gleno-humeral shoulder flexion, the stationary arm of the goniometer would be positioned where?

    A. Parallel to the humerus

    B. Medial aspect of the ulna

    C. Longitudinal axis of the radius

    D. Parallel to the lateral midline of the trunk

6. The *most* important goal in teaching ADLs to a patient with LE, above knee amputation is:

    A. Use of adaptive equipment

    B. How to supervise others who help with home management

    C. Energy conservation and work simplification

    D. Cognitive retraining

7. A rotator cuff injury would result in clinical features that include:

    A. No restrictions in AROM of the shoulder

    B. Painful arch 50 to 100 degrees and restricted AROM in shoulder abduction and flexion

    C. Total restriction in AROM of the shoulder

    D. Only full PROM would indicate restrictions

Use the following information to answer questions 8 and 9: During a coping skills activity in an inpatient psychiatric unit, your patient suddenly starts sweating, complains of his heart pounding, feels dizzy, and fears he is losing control. He suddenly runs out of the group.

8. These symptoms *most* likely describe:
    A. Generalized anxiety
    B. A heart attack
    C. Panic attack
    D. Stress

9. The OT's *best* initial response would be:
    A. Encourage the patient to return
    B. Notify other team members
    C. Remain with the group members
    D. Check on patient directly

10. When testing scapula elevation, which two muscles would be palpated?
    A. The rhomboids
    B. Sternocleidomastoid and upper trapezius
    C. Upper trapezius and levator scapula
    D. Pectoralis major and minor

11. The certification exam for the OTA is:
    A. The same as the OT exam but OTAs have more time
    B. Different from the OT exam
    C. The same as the OT exam but easier to pass
    D. The same as the OT but given on different days

12. Ataxia results in a lack of postural stability. If a client can ambulate but has ataxia and fatigue, what would you recommend while preparing meals in the kitchen?
    A. A home program of postural stability exercises
    B. Energy conservation and work simplification education
    C. The client should use a wheelchair in the kitchen
    D. A home health aide should take care of meal preparation

13. Spinal reflexes are considered to be more primitive and are noted for their quick action and extinction. They include all of the following *except*:
    A. Flexor withdrawal
    B. Extensor thrust
    C. Positive supporting reaction
    D. Neck righting

14. What do the initials MBO stand for?
    A. Management, bettered, outcomes
    B. Manager, believed, outcomes
    C. Management, by, objective
    D. Manager, bought, outcomes

15. When an elderly patient is ready for discharge from an acute hospital, equipment for home must be considered. Medicare covers durable medical equipment, which is defined as all of the following *except:*
    A. Can withstand repeated use
    B. The cost is set by Medicare
    C. Is primarily for medical purposes
    D. Is not useful in absence of illness or injury

16. Culture can have an impact on behavior. The development of suspiciousness and paranoid ideas is *most* commonly found in which of the following populations?
    A. Immigrants
    B. African-Americans
    C. Caucasians
    D. Native Americans

17. Your client is a 12-month-old girl who exhibits poor integration of primitive reflexes with impaired hand-to-mouth and hand-to-body movements. What would be the *best* intervention by occupational therapy?
    A. Rolling, pushing up on extended elbows from a prone position
    B. Visual tracking of a toy to increase eye ROM
    C. Reaching for a toy to improve eye-hand coordination
    D. Moving small pegs from cup to cup

18. The theory that incorporates diagonal patterns, manual contacts, and distinct verbal and tactile cues is:
    A. Rood
    B. Proprioceptive neuromuscular facilitation (PNF)
    C. Brunnstrom
    D. Bobath

19. The directive group was developed by Kathy Kaplan. It may be described as all of the following *except:*
    A. It is based on the model of human occupation
    B. It is designed for higher functioning patients
    C. Group leaders are active and supportive
    D. Groups are often co-led

20. The president of AOTA is:
    A. Elected by the representative assembly
    B. Elected by the AOTA members
    C. Appointed by the AOTA executive director
    D. Last year's vice president

21. How many degrees of freedom of motion are available at the hip joint?
    A. One
    B. Two
    C. Three
    D. Four

22. Which of the following statements is *not* true about delirium?
    A. Delirium is a disease
    B. Mood, perception, and behavior may be abnormal
    C. Causes include CNS disease, systemic disease, intoxication, or withdrawal from substances
    D. The neuroanatomical area affected is the reticular formation

23. Which of the following activities is the *best* choice for a client with dissociative disorder whose goal is to increase her self-understanding and to express her feelings?
    A. Horticulture
    B. Arts and crafts
    C. Sports
    D. Art therapy

24. The collateral ligaments of the MP joints are taut in:
    A. Flexion
    B. Extension
    C. Abduction
    D. Adduction

25. The muscular pad created by intrinsic muscles to the fifth digit is known as the:
    A. Thenar eminence
    B. Hypothenar eminence
    C. Palmar crease
    D. Palmar arch

26. A patient diagnosed with Alzheimer's disease is about to be discharged to his home. A critical occupational therapy goal at this time should include:
    A. Increase level of activity
    B. Education of client
    C. Education of caregiver
    D. Increase memory aids

27. The *most* important area of occupational therapy intervention for a person with LE, above knee amputation is:
    A. Adaptive equipment assessment
    B. Instruction in donning and doffing the prosthetic device
    C. Gait training
    D. Teaching the client skin inspection of the stump

28. *The Practice Framework* includes:
    A. Occupational performance areas, performance skills, and performance patterns
    B. Definitions of current frames of reference
    C. Suggestions for documentation methods, including SOAP and POMR
    D. Budget guidelines for OT departments

29. What nerve passes through the carpal tunnel?
    A. Median
    B. Ulnar
    C. Radial
    D. Musculocutaneous

30. The end feel is the sensation transmitted to the therapist's hands at the extreme end of PROM and indicates the structures that limit joint movement. A soft end feel is:

    A. Firm, from a soft tissue stretch

    B. Abrupt, with a hard stop to the movement

    C. Soft, from a soft tissue opposition

    D. Capsular, like stretching a piece of leather

31. Which of the following causes of dementia is reversible?

    A. Alzheimer's
    B. Vascular disease
    C. AIDS
    D. Depression

32. The accreditation committee of AOTA is responsible for the approval of:

    A. Certification of OTAs and the registration of OTs

    B. Occupational therapy educational programs

    C. Licensure in states

    D. Policies in AOTA

Use the following information to answer questions 33 and 34: Another occupational therapist has told you during lunch that she is really behind in her billable units for the week so she is going to bill patients for the time this week and make up for it next week.

33. This breaks what section of the AOTA code of ethics?

    A. Principle 1, beneficence

    B. Principle 3, autonomy, privacy, and confidentiality

    C. Principle 5, justice

    D. Principle 6, veracity

34. The *best* response to this situation is:

    A. Notify the billing department that false billing has occurred

    B. Notify the area coordinator that there is a problem in the department

    C. Speak to the therapist privately and tell her that this is unethical

    D. Report the unethical behavior to the ethics committee of AOTA

35. When evaluating a client with an orthopedic condition, which frame of reference is *best*?
    A. Sensory motor
    B. Cognitive
    C. Developmental
    D. Biomechanical

36. The *best* group activity designed specifically for the chronically mentally ill patient who has difficulty with motor planning, verbalization, and eye contact is:

    A. Tennis

    B. Basketball

    C. Walking

    D. Parachute games

37. A homonymous hemianopsia is a loss of visual field secondary to a CVA. What would be the visual loss for a right CVA?

    A. Right nasal side and temporal side of both the right and left eyes

    B. Right nasal side of right eye only

    C. Left nasal side of right eye and left temporal side of left eye

    D. Left nasal side of left eye only

38. If a client's UE is extremely difficult to move and PROM is impossible, the muscle tone would be:

    A. Athetoid

    B. Flaccid

    C. Spastic

    D. Ataxic

39. The OT shows a group of children several items on a table. While the children close their eyes, the OT removes one item. The children open their eyes and guess which item is missing. Which of the following goals is *most* developed by the children?

    A. Increase eye-hand coordination

    B. Increase bilateral integration

    C. Increase form constancy

    D. Increase visual memory

40. Social smiling in infancy can be elicited by the mother at what age?

    A. 1 to 2 weeks

    B. 2 to 4 weeks

    C. 4 to 8 weeks

    D. 16 weeks

41. Medicare will pay for all of the following *except:*

    A. Trapeze

    B. Splints

    C. Bedside commode

    D. Grab bars

42. An adult with schizophrenia can be diagnosed from all of the following symptoms *except:*

    A. Social dysfunction

    B. Delusions

    C. Disorganized speech

    D. Substance abuse

43. The World Federation of Occupational Therapists (WFOT) is:

    A. Composed of NBCOT-registered OTs who work overseas

    B. Managed by AOTA

    C. Composed of OTs from around the world

    D. Part of your membership from AOTA

44. Facilitation of patient acceptance of an amputation is often addressed by occupational therapy. What is the *most* important area addressed to encourage acceptance of the prosthetic device?

    A. Patient's acceptance of new body image

    B. Patient's ability to deny or express anger

    C. Patient's ability to accept dependence

    D. Patient's ability to use adaptive equipment with the prosthetic device

Use the following information to answer questions 45 and 46: A parent complains to the OT that her 6-year-old child does not listen to her when she tells him to be quiet in church and stop bothering other people.

45. The OT recognizes the child's behavior as:

    A. Negativism

    B. Symbolization

    C. Egocentrism

    D. Imminent justice

46. The *best* response the OT could give to the mother is:

    A. Ignore the child's behavior

    B. Educate the parents to normal development

    C. Talk to the child about his behavior

    D. To redirect the child's attention to something else

47. The *most* common hallucination for patients with schizophrenia is:

    A. Visual

    B. Auditory

    C. Tactile

    D. Olfactory

48. The *best* example of an activity that uses Allen's cognitive disability frame of reference is:

    A. Leather lacing a wallet

    B. Discussion group

    C. Movement or dance therapy

    D. Draw a person

49. Medicare will pay for durable medical equipment if it meets the criteria and is ordered by a physician. A physician's order must include all of the following *except:*

    A. Estimated cost

    B. Diagnosis

    C. Prognosis

    D. Reason for need

50. An OT is performing a COTE assessment on a 15-year-old male patient who is feeling depressed. He stops his activity after 2 to 3 minutes and tells the therapist that he is "too tired" to continue. The OT hypothesizes that he has difficulty with:

    A. Reality orientation

    B. Initiating activity

    C. Responsibility

    D. Problem solving

Section Seven Answers and Explanations

1. Answer: C
This is the hallmark sign for delirium versus dementia. Dementia is a syndrome that includes cognitive impairments without impairment in consciousness.

2. Answer: B
A significant issue for people with substance dependency is organizing a social network that is supportive. Since substance abuse often becomes the primary focus of activity, a significant OT goal is time management and the restructuring of social activities to prevent slippage. A and D can also be helpful.

3. Answer: A
Infancy is considered from 0 to 18 months and ends when the child is able to speak. Creeping occurs at about 40 weeks. Climbing stairs occurs around 2 years. Bowel control occurs around 3 years.

4. Answer: B
AOTF's primary goal is the development of research in occupational therapy. In addition, AOTF provides scholarships, fundraising, and houses the occupational therapy library.

5. Answer: D
The movable arm is parallel to the humerus midline. B and C are not involved.

6. Answer: C
People with amputations spend more energy during ADLs than people without amputations. Adaptive equipment might help, however, energy conservation is first. Supervising others and cognitive retraining are only appropriate if there are deficiencies in these areas.

7. Answer: B
There would be loss of AROM. The supraspinatus assists with shoulder abduction. Other muscles would compensate to allow some movement. PROM is usually normal in rotator cuff injuries.

8. Answer: C
Panic attacks have a sudden onset that can reach a peak within 10 minutes. Other signs include trembling, sensation of shortness of breath, feeling of choking, chest pain, nausea, derealization, fear of dying, paralysis, and chills. Generalized anxiety is chronic and persistent. It is always possible that the patient might be having a heart attack and should be checked. Stress is a generalized term.

9. Answer: D
Safety of the patient is always the first priority. While other responses are relevant, the initial responsibility is to secure the patient.

10. Answer: C
Upper trapezius and levator scapula are the primary movers for scapula elevation. Rhomboids assist when the trapezius is weak. The sternocleidomastoid flexes the neck. The pectoralis minor can act as a downward rotator of the scapula.

11. Answer: B
The certification exam for the OTA is completely different from the exam for the OT.

12. Answer: B
Energy conservation and work simplification are the priorities after safety and might lead to adaptive equipment. Although balance enhancement exercises would be helpful, the fatigue must be addressed first. A home health aide might be helpful but would reduce the client's sense of independence and increase the feeling of loss of self-control.

13. Answer: D
Neck righting is an upper brainstem induced reflex indicating a refined postural adjustment. Flexor withdrawal, extensor thrust, and positive supporting reaction are all spinal reflexes.

14. Answer: C

Management by objective is a common approach to managing occupational therapy departments and other health care programs.

15. Answer: B

Medicare does not assign the cost of equipment, however, it is expected that the cost will be comparable to local costs for that item. Durable medical equipment paid for under Medicare must withstand repeated use, be used for medical purposes, and be useless in absence of illness or injury.

16. Answer: A

There is no significant increase in paranoid ideas in the following cultural groups: African-Americans, Caucasians, or Native Americans. Recent immigrants have a higher rate of developing delusional disorder due to the uncertainty of their new environment. Immigrants must adjust to new people with different mannerisms, responses, and language.

17. Answer: A

Although other areas of intervention would be valuable, working on integration of primitive reflexes will enhance overall development. Visual tracking and eye-hand coordination can be addressed after the reflexes. Small pegs are too difficult and dangerous for any 1-year-old.

18. Answer: B

PNF is a classic movement treatment approach developed in the late 1940s. PNF uses the theory of diagonal or spinal movement as essential for motor control and the basis for normal movement. Rood uses a developmental sequence as a prerequisite for recovery. Icing and brush are Rood techniques. Brunnstrom focuses on synergy status and the stages of recovery. Bobath places emphasis on reflex inhibiting postures (RIP) and key point of control.

19. Answer: B

The directive group is designed for patients with minimal functioning who are often excluded from traditional group treatment. A, C, and D are true of a directive group.

20. Answer: B

The president of AOTA is elected by the members. The president is a volunteer position unlike the executive director of AOTA.

21. Answer: C

The hip is a ball and socket joint that allows flexion/extension, rotation, and abduction/adduction.

22. Answer: A

Delirium is a syndrome, not a disease. Delirium has many causes that result in a pattern of symptoms. These symptoms include impairment in consciousness and cognitive deficits. Neurological signs include tremor, nystagmus, incoordination, and urinary incontinence.

23. Answer: D

Expressive arts such as art, dance, movement, and writing are excellent resources to increase a patient's understanding of her dynamics and related feelings. A, B, and C are task-oriented modalities.

24. Answer: A

Collateral ligaments are designed to be taut in flexion to check the movement of the digits at the joint. They act as a stability function.

25. Answer: B

The muscles of the hand form two masses in the palm. These are the thenar at the base of the thumb and the hypothenar eminence at the base of the little finger.

26. Answer: C

Although A, B, and D are relevant in the initial treatment stage, the OT should shift focus to the caregiver at discharge. Since this is a progressive disorder, the caregivers should be prepared for emerging deficits. The OT can learn from the caregiver about the patient's individual needs to customize the discharge plan.

27. Answer: D

Skin breakdown is common, especially for people with LEAK amputation. Often skin breakdown is caused by poor socket fit or wrinkles in the stump sock. Adaptive equipment and donning training are important after the priority of skin care. Gait training will likely be addressed by physical therapy with OT assisting in safety issues.

28. Answer: A

The Practice Framework is an official document of AOTA and defines the practice of occupational therapy. In addition, this document addresses context, activity demands, and client factors.

29. Answer: A

Carpal tunnel syndrome involves the median nerve.

30. Answer: C

A soft end feel is compression of tissue and feels soft, not firm, abrupt, or capsular. A and B are not pathological; D is an abnormal condition.

31. Answer: D

Dementia from Alzheimer's, vascular disease, and AIDS is not reversible. Depression in the elderly is often confused with dementia because the patient presents with confusion and memory impairment. Also known as pseudodementia, this depression is most likely treatable and reversible.

32. Answer: B

All OT and OTA educational programs must maintain accreditation with AOTA. Programs without accreditation cannot have their graduates take the registration exam. Without taking the exam, graduates are unable to practice occupational therapy.

33. Answer: D

Documentation is covered by the code of ethics under communication that contains false, fraudulent, deceptive, or unfair statements (AOTA, 2004).

34. Answer: C

The first action is to speak to the therapist who made the comment. Although it may be uncomfortable, as an occupational therapist it is your duty to stop an unethical practice. If the therapist continues with the plan to bill ahead, speak to a supervisor. If the supervisor does not stop the practice, report the information to the standards and ethics committee (SEC) of AOTA. The SEC will provide you with information and support on how to handle the problem. Ethical problems are always difficult to address, but as an OT you have a high standard to protect your consumers.

35. Answer: D

The biomechanical frame of reference (FOR) looks at forces affecting function. Orthopedic conditions use MMT, goniometry, and strength training to improve function. Kinematics is inherent in this intervention, therefore, the biomechanical FOR is appropriate. Sensory motor FOR is generally employed when CNS damage has occurred. Cognitive and developmental FOR are not appropriate for orthopedic conditions, as the therapist can assume that no cognitive or development issues are present as primary issues in treatment.

36. Answer: D

Parachute games provide noncompetitive sensorimotor activity. Researchers theorize that perceptual, posture, body image, and motor planning deficits found in patients with schizophrenia are the result of poor sensory integration. Tennis and basketball are competitive. Walking is unstructured and not as stimulating as parachute games.

37. Answer: C

The right CVA with left involved extremities would have a hemianopsia of the left nasal side of the right eye and the left temporal side of the left eye.

38. Answer: C

Spasticity is a condition of hypertonia. Athetoid is associated with hypotonia. The client would have full PROM but decreased coordination. Flaccid muscles are seen in extreme hypotonia. Ataxia is also within the hypotonic range with decreased coordination and controlled movement.

39. Answer: D
While other goals can be integrated, visual memory is primary to the game.

40. Answer: C
Social smiling occurs between 4 to 8 weeks. Infant smiles are endogenous and apparent in blind infants as well as sighted infants. Visual fixation occurs between 2 to 4 weeks. Spontaneous social smiling is evident at 16 weeks.

41. Answer: D
Medicare will pay for a trapeze if used by someone confined to bed and is needed for mobility. Medicare will pay for a splint if used to increase or restore function. Medicare will pay for a bedside commode if used by someone confined to a room. Medicare will not pay for grab bars because these are considered self-help items.

42. Answer: D
The disturbance cannot be due to direct physiological effects of a substance. Social dysfunction, delusions, and disorganized speech are among the symptoms needed to diagnose someone with schizophrenia. Other symptoms include hallucinations, negative symptoms, occupational dysfunction, and grossly disorganized or catatonic behavior. Negative symptoms include flat affect, alogia, and avolition.

43. Answer: C
The WFOT is composed of OTs around the world. Members do not have to be AOTA registered; however, therapists can pay their WFOT dues when they pay their AOTA dues.

44. Answer: A
Acceptance facilitation is an important role for occupational therapy. The OT can do this in conjunction with the prosthesis training. Anger can be addressed in acceptance. Independence instead of dependency is the goal of OT. Adaptive equipment will help in all areas of acceptance but must be appropriately timed.

45. Answer: C
Piaget defines egocentrism as behavior typical of 2- to 7-year-olds in the stage of pre-operational thought. Children in this stage feel they are the center of the universe, have a limited point of view, and are not capable of empathizing with others. A child at this stage is not being negativistic. Symbolization is the ability of an infant to create an image of an object. Imminent justice is the belief that punishment for wrongdoing is inevitable.

46. Answer: B
Because the child is not doing anything wrong, educating the parent is the most supportive. Although redirecting the child may stop the behavior, the best response is parent education.

47. Answer: B
Hearing voices is the most common hallucination in schizophrenia, with visual as second most common. Visual hallucinations alone are more common with people in detoxification programs for drugs and alcohol. Tactile and olfactory hallucinations are less common.

48. Answer: A
The wallet includes the most steps in reasoning, decision making, problem solving, and performance. A discussion group is open-ended and unstructured. A movement or dance group usually includes aspects of sensorimotor or projective arts. Drawing a person is typical of the psychoanalytic frame of reference.

49. Answer: A
Medicare requires a durable medical equipment prescription from a physician to include the diagnosis, prognosis, reason for need, and estimation for the length of need. The cost does not need to be included in the order.

50. Answer: B
Common symptoms of depression are decreased pleasure or interest in activities, fatigue, and decreased energy. Reality orientation is awareness of person, place, and time. There is no indication of this problem. Responsibility and problem solving cannot be judged due to limited data. Further assessment is needed.

Section Eight

1. An OT consulting to a long-term care facility should do all of the following *except*:
   A. Provide input on selection of forms and the documentation process
   B. Keep activity personnel apprised of changes in regulations
   C. Suggest ways staff can do physical therapy activities to cover the lack of PTs
   D. Advise on enhancement of group dynamics and resident involvement

2. Universal precautions help prevent transmission of HIV and hepatitis B. The body fluids that universal precautions apply to include:
   A. Blood and other fluids containing blood
   B. Feces and urine
   C. Sweat
   D. Tears

3. A teenage girl with muscular dystrophy wants to apply her own make-up. As her occupational therapist, you recommend all of the following *except*:
   A. Prop elbow on the table to save energy
   B. Groom in phases with rest breaks
   C. Take a long shower before starting
   D. Enlarge the handles on the make-up items

4. At 40 weeks of age, a child is approximately capable of all of the following *except*:
   A. Sitting alone
   B. Creeping
   C. Ability to say one word
   D. Feeling shame

5. JCAHO accredits health care facilities. What do the initials stand for?
   A. Joint Commission on Accreditation of Healthcare Organizations
   B. Joint Committee for Accreditation of Hospital Operations
   C. Joint Consensus on Accreditation of Healthcare Operations
   D. Joint Caregivers for Accreditation of Hospital Organization

6. In a stressful situation, the function of the sympathetic branch of the autonomic nervous system is all of the following *except*:
   A. Increase heart rate and force of contraction
   B. Pupils of the eyes dilate
   C. Increase sweat
   D. Contract the pupils of the eye, decrease secretions of the salivary glands

7. Persons with AIDS are prone to opportunistic diseases. Which of the following is *not* likely to be seen in a person with AIDS?
   A. Amyotrophic lateral sclerosis
   B. Kaposi's sarcoma
   C. Pneumocystic carinii pneumonia
   D. Toxoplasmosis

8. The science of workplace design is called:
   A. Workspace planning
   B. Accessibility planning
   C. Work hardening
   D. Ergonomics

9. A client who wants to use a computer but only has gross motor hand movement would use what type of input device?
   A. Standard keyboard
   B. Expanded keyboard
   C. Joystick
   D. Single switch

10. During a home visit with a young mother who recently injured herself in a fall, you overhear her husband hitting their son repeatedly upstairs. Your client begins to cry and suddenly appears frightened. She asks you to leave because she does not want her husband to see you. What should you do?
    A. Leave as you are told
    B. Ignore the incident until further proof
    C. Run upstairs to stop the beating
    D. Secure the safety of the patient and report the abuse to authorities

11. Chronic obstructive pulmonary disease (COPD) refers to all diseases that cause irreversible damage to the lungs. For the patient with COPD, all of the following activities are consistently difficult *except*:
    A. Decision making
    B. Eating
    C. Speaking
    D. Exercise

12. A young, healthy adult younger than age 40 will have blood pressure of less than:
    A. 120/80
    B. 130/90
    C. 140/80
    D. 140/90

13. A child must be able to identify body positioning in space and realize the course of movement to change his or her position to another position. This awareness of space direction will directly affect which of the following?
    A. Sorting one body part to another
    B. Reading and writing from left to right
    C. Picking an object out against a background
    D. Drawing a person

14. When speaking to a person with a hearing impairment, the OT should do all of the following *except:*
    A. Keep hands away from your face
    B. Speak slower
    C. Talk face to face
    D. Get the person's attention before starting to speak

15. Tracing one's body on a sheet of paper is *most* useful with what type of psychiatric disorder?
    A. Major depression
    B. Eating disorder
    C. Schizophrenia, paranoid type
    D. Bipolar, manic phase

16. Which of the following activities is the *best* initial choice for a patient in an acute paranoid state?
    A. Cooking group
    B. Reading a newspaper
    C. Organizing a daily schedule
    D. Arts and crafts

17. Which is *not* true of multiple sclerosis?
    A. It is a slowly progressive disease of the central nervous system
    B. It is characterized by demyelination of nerves
    C. Symptoms have exacerbations and remissions
    D. The onset of the disease is most common between ages 3 to 8

18. What is the *best* treatment for an adult with a head injury at Rancho Los Amigos level I or II?
    A. Community re-entry activities
    B. A functional task such as making a sandwich
    C. A simple task such as painting a birdhouse with one color
    D. PROM and graded sensory stimulation

19. Vegetative signs in depression include all of the following *except*:
    A. Psychomotor retardation
    B. Obsessive ruminations
    C. Weight loss
    D. Abnormal menses

20. Which of the following statements is *not* true regarding ECT treatments?
    A. Commonly used for major depressive disorder
    B. Patient experiences no movement during treatment
    C. Appearance of gooseflesh is noted
    D. A secondary stimulus may be needed to induce a seizure

21. What age group has a normal pulse rate of 115 to 130 beats per minute?
    A. First year after birth
    B. Childhood years
    C. Adult years
    D. Later years

22. Can an adult be first diagnosed with mental retardation?
    A. Yes, but only if there is a previous history of mental retardation from birth
    B. Yes, even without a history of mental retardation
    C. Yes, but only if another psychiatric diagnosis can be found
    D. No, only children can be diagnosed with mental retardation

23. Rehabilitative or educational technologies include all of the following *except:*
    A. Prosthesis
    B. Cognitive rehabilitation software
    C. Biofeedback
    D. Functional electrical stimulation

24. Which of the following OT groups is the *best* choice for a patient who is abusing substances and has a poor self-concept?
    A. Arts and crafts
    B. Cooking
    C. Shopping
    D. Life management

25. Activities such as slow, rhythmic rocking; deep breathing; and mental imagery are relevant choices for what type of OT group?
    A. Leisure skills
    B. Value clarification
    C. Stress management
    D. Weight management

26. Good skin techniques are important for children with spina bifida. These techniques include all of the following *except:*
    A. Thick and deep padding
    B. Check skin for pressure sores
    C. Change positions frequently
    D. Avoid tight-fitting clothes

27. All of the following counseling techniques are appropriate to use with a newly admitted patient *except:*
    A. Confrontation
    B. Empathy
    C. Concreteness
    D. Respect

28. A person with restricted ROM throughout the UE would *best* benefit from what adaptive equipment?
    A. Extended or lengthened handles of eating utensils
    B. Rocker knife
    C. Built-up handles
    D. Spill-proof cup

29. Which of the following is *not* true of attention deficit disorder?
    A. More boys are affected than girls
    B. Children are of average or above average intelligence
    C. Children have fair to good problem-solving skills
    D. Symptoms might include impulsiveness

30. In the elderly, age-related changes such as gait, postural instability, decreased vision, decreased hearing, and forgetfulness all increase the risk of what?
    A. Drug dependence
    B. Falls
    C. Loneliness
    D. Entering a nursing home

31. What defense is your patient using when he tells you he sent his wife roses after a physical fight with her?
    A. Projection
    B. Undoing
    C. Splitting
    D. Passive-aggressive

32. Joint protection techniques include all of the following *except*:
    A. Maintain joints in correct position
    B. Use hands instead of shoulders
    C. Bend hips and knees but keep back straight
    D. Distribute load over two or more joints

33. When is anxiety considered pathological?
    A. When intensity does not match the situation
    B. When it accompanies something new
    C. When considering one's identity
    D. When facing an illness

34. A fracture in a diseased or weakened bone that has been subjected to a normal strain is called:
    A. Greenstick fracture
    B. Pathological fracture
    C. Compound fracture
    D. Comminuted fracture

35. How should flammable arts and craft supplies such as paint, stain, cleaners, and thinners be stored in the OT clinic?
    A. In a locked closet
    B. In an open area, supervised by staff
    C. In a ventilated metal cabinet
    D. In a room with a sink and water

36. Ankylosing spondylitis can result in a rigid spinal column with flexion and rotation of the trunk severely restricted. What ADL task would be *most* difficult for this patient?
    A. Bathing
    B. Donning shoes and socks
    C. Feeding self
    D. Meal preparation

37. What type of disease is rheumatoid arthritis?
    A. A degenerative joint disease
    B. An inflammatory joint disease
    C. A disease seen only in the elderly population
    D. A joint disease that affects the large diarthrodial joints only

38. A 46-year-old male comes to you complaining of diffuse left elbow pain. His elbow becomes stiff when he picks things up with his left hand and the pain in his left hand increases. What frame of reference would you use to treat his lateral epicondylitis?
    A. Model of human occupation
    B. Acquisitional
    C. Biomechanical
    D. Developmental

39. Why is it important to ask a patient about his or her hobbies, lifestyle, and occupations in relationship to hand use?
    A. To help establish patient rapport
    B. A repetitive pattern of use may become apparent
    C. To see if the patient has a good balance of activities in his or her life
    D. To suggest a job change before you examine the hand

40. Which evaluation is *best* to measure developmental skills in a pediatric population?
    A. Southern California Sensory Integration Tests (SCSIT)
    B. Motor-Free Visual Perception Test (MVPT)
    C. Miller Assessment for Preschoolers (MAP)
    D. Play Skills Inventory

41. Tri-Alliance is:
    A. A health insurance program for people in the military services
    B. A program of AOTA
    C. Special research of OTs and primates
    D. A mouthpiece to use on a computer

42. Medicare Part B is:
    A. Supplementary medical insurance
    B. Available to all U. S. citizens
    C. Free to those age 65 and over
    D. Not available to those people with end-stage renal disease

43. When a patient falls in the clinic, the *first* thing that should be done after ensuring the patient's safety and well-being is:
    A. File an incident report following the facility's policies
    B. Call the family and let them know
    C. Take the patient's temperature and blood pressure
    D. Notify the next shift of the problem

44. Evaluating a patient begins:
    A. As soon as the patient walks (or is wheeled) into the clinic
    B. When performing AROM to observe limitations
    C. While reading the medical referral
    D. While making small talk with the patient prior to testing PROM

45. Precautions for dysphagia patients include all of the following *except:*
    A. After feeding, the patient should remain upright for 20 minutes to prevent aspiration
    B. If food remains in the mouth after feeding, have the patient wash it down with a drink
    C. Do not schedule eating sessions after strenuous activity
    D. Do not use foods with nuts, fibers, or extreme spices that are difficult to chew

46. While conducting an ADL evaluation, your patient with schizophrenia conveys very little information and tends to respond vaguely to your questions. This speech disturbance is known as:
    A. Dysarthria
    B. Pressured speech
    C. Poverty of speech
    D. Poverty of content of speech

47. Which is *not* one of the general cognitive changes considered to be part of the normal aging process?
    A. Loss of brain cells
    B. Impaired thought processes
    C. Temporary decrease in mental function following an acute illness
    D. Ability to solve practical problems in daily living

48. All of the following are effective in reducing hand edema for the post surgery client *except:*
    A. Cold, wet packs
    B. Massage
    C. Elevation
    D. Isotoner brand gloves

49. What type of spoon should be used to feed a child with reflex biting?
    A. A traditional teaspoon for normal eating
    B. A traditional soup spoon to hold more food
    C. A narrow, shallow, firm plastic- or rubber-coated spoon
    D. A square-shaped spade spoon with open front

50. While working with a patient who is post myocardial infarction, activities should be stopped when all of the following signs are present *except:*
    A. Dyspnea
    B. Palpitations
    C. Pulse between 95 to 110
    D. Glassy stare

Section Eight Answers and Explanations

1. Answer: C
PT is out of the expertise of both the facility staff and the OT. A, B, and D are all roles of the consulting OT.

2. Answer: A
Universal precautions should be applied to blood and other fluids containing blood. Feces, urine, sweat, and tears have extremely low to nonexistent rates of HIV infection unless they include blood. Universal precautions include gloves, gowns, face guards, and cleaning with bleach and water. The therapist may choose to wear gloves when treating all patients to reduce spreading germs to others. Washing hands before and after all treatment is good general practice.

3. Answer: C
Taking a long shower before applying make-up may be too exhausting. Energy conservation is the priority for this teenager. A, B, and D will all help conserve energy.

4. Answer: D
At approximately 12 to 18 months, children can show various emotions such as distress, anger, fear, sadness, and shame. At 3 to 4 years they can feel guilt. Sitting alone, creeping, and saying one word are all developmentally appropriate landmarks for 40 weeks.

5. Answer: A
The initials JCAHO stand for the Joint Commission on Accreditation of Healthcare Organizations.

6. Answer: D
Increased heart rate, dilated pupils, and increased salivary secretions are all sympathetic.

7. Answer: A
People with AIDS are prone to Kaposi's sarcoma, pneumocystic carinii pneumonia, and toxoplasmosis. Amyotrophic lateral sclerosis is a neurological disorder with onset between 40 to 70 years old.

8. Answer: D
Ergonomics is the science of workplace design.

9. Answer: D
A single switch is for a person with only gross hand movements. Keyboards and joysticks require finger gross motor or some fine motor.

10. Answer: D
State laws vary, however, the OT is usually mandated to report the incident to the appropriate authority. Most states have a department of family services, which is responsible for investigating suspected abusive situations. If you are not sure who to call, ask your local police department for the child protection agency phone number.

11. Answer: A
Decision making is difficult for a person with COPD only if the blood gases are off. Eating, speaking, and exercising are always difficult, if not impossible.

12. Answer: D
The medical community is currently discussing whether to lower the definition of "normal" blood pressure. Generally, the medical community defined high blood pressure for an adult as 140/90 or higher and 160/90 as high for a person over age 40. Some medical doctors prefer 120/80 as normal and are more likely to give the diagnosis of hypertension if higher. The therapist should consult with the medical doctor to the ideal blood pressure of each client.

13. Answer: B
A child's awareness of space and direction helps him or her read left to right and place words on paper. Sorting and drawing represents body image, which begins during infancy. Picking objects out is an example of figure ground.

14. Answer: B

Speak at a normal speed, tone, and volume. Keep hands away from your face, get the person's attention before starting, and talk face to face.

15. Answer: B

Body image is a major aspect of OT treatment for people with eating disorders. Body image is intact for people with major depression. People with schizophrenia or bipolar disorder may find this activity too threatening.

16. Answer: C

Setting a daily routine will offer a sense of control, security, and predictability. Cooking groups and crafts require multiple steps and interaction with others. The newspaper may be too stimulating and open ended.

17. Answer: D

The onset of the disease is 16 to 40 years old. A, B, and C are all true.

18. Answer: D

A Rancho Los Amigos (RLA) level of I or II means the patient appears to be sleeping or is awake but nonresponsive. PROM and sensory stimulation are appropriate treatments. A simple task is appropriate for level IV as long as it is safe, as these patients are easily agitated. Making a sandwich is a good task for level V. Community re-entry activities are best for levels VI and above.

19. Answer: B

Vegetative signs refer to functions related to the autonomic nervous system. Obsessive rumination is a tense state of mind related to thought content. A, C, and D are vegetative signs.

20. Answer: B

The first behavioral sign of ECT is a slight plantar extension of the feet followed by some toe, finger, or other movement.

21. Answer: A

Children from birth to 1 year old have normal pulse rates of 115 to 130. The childhood years are normal at 80 to 115. Adult years are 72 to 80 and later years are 60 to 72.

22. Answer: A

Adults can be diagnosed with mental retardation. Almost always the adult was diagnosed as a young child and carries the diagnosis into adulthood. A child or adult cannot be diagnosed with mental retardation unless born with it. Mental retardation is not a diagnosis that can be given to a child who once had normal intelligence.

23. Answer: A

A prosthesis is considered assistive or adaptive technology, not rehabilitative or educational technology. B, C, and D are all rehabilitative or educational technologies.

24. Answer: D

Arts and crafts, cooking, and shopping are problem-solving tasks. Decision making is a primary goal. A secondary effect may lead to increased self-esteem. Life management includes coping skills and self-control. These contribute to improving one's self-concept.

25. Answer: C

These are all effective OT techniques used in stress management leading to relaxation.

26. Answer: A

Thick padding often adds more pressure to the skin. Padding should only be the absolute minimum for comfort.

27. Answer: A

Confrontation is a skill used once rapport and trust have been established. It serves to point out discrepancies between thought and behavior. Empathy is the skill of fully communicating understanding of a patient's needs and feelings. Concreteness is the skill of seeking clarification, often using open-ended questions. Respect is the skill of communicating professional concern with a nonjudgmental tone.

28. Answer: A

An extended handle on the eating utensils would allow the person to feed himself or herself without moving the UE as much as traditional utensils require. A rocker knife is best used for one hand functioning. Built-up handles are best used by people with grasp problems. A spill-proof cup is best used by someone with tremors.

29. Answer: C

Children with attention deficit disorder (ADD) are more likely to be boys, have average or above average intelligence, and be impulsive. Some have hyperactivity (ADHD) as well. Children with ADD frequently have poor problem-solving skills.

30. Answer: B

The term "risk" suggests a negative component among the choices. Falling is the number one problem among the elderly and is related to normal changes, pathological changes, and the environment.

31. Answer: B

Undoing is the act of taking a positive action to counter an act perceived by one's ego as threatening. This is commonly seen in patients with obsessive-compulsive disorder. Projection is attributing feelings onto someone or something else, common in patients who are paranoid. Splitting is dividing people into bad or good categories, common in patients with borderline personality. Passive-aggressive is anger turned against the self.

32. Answer: B

Joint protection includes palms instead of fingers and shoulders instead of hands. Use the load carrying muscles and joints over the fine motor muscles and joints.

33. Answer: A

Pathological anxiety is an inappropriate response to a stressor in intensity or duration. B, C, and D are all normal anxiety.

34. Answer: B

A pathological fracture can indicate a tumor or osteoporosis. A greenstick fracture is seen in immature bones of children. A compound fracture is a bone broken in several places, and a comminuted fracture is a crush injury.

35. Answer: C

All flammable supplies should be kept in a ventilated, locked, metal cabinet unless the label warns differently. Hazardous materials must be used and disposed of following strict regulations. Most facilities have a hazardous waste management supervisor. Check with this person concerning supplies and consider nontoxic alternatives.

36. Answer: B

Dressing the LE is the most problematic.

37. Answer: B

Rheumatoid arthritis (RA) is a classic connective tissue disease because of the inflammatory process and systemic involvement. Degenerative joint disease is non-inflammatory, usually associated with osteoarthritis. RA is noted in both young and older populations and in both large and small joints.

38. Answer: C

Biomechanical frame of reference is best because of the orthopedic nature of the injury and the patient's complaint.

39. Answer: B

Good history taking may show a pattern of repetitive injury. Rapport building is important also but secondary to the nature of hand injuries. A good balance of activities and possible job changes comes later in treatment.

40. Answer: C

The MAP is a developmental assessment. The SCSIT is an evaluation of sensory integration. The MVPT is an assessment tool for visual perception with children ages 4 to 8. The Play Skills Inventory addresses observed play habits.

41. Answer: A

Tri-Alliance is a health insurance plan for military personnel and their families. AOTA does have an alliance with the PT and speech associations, however, A is the better answer. C and D are not true.

42. Answer: A

Medicare Part B is supplementary medical insurance to Part A. It is available to persons over 65 and those with disabilities for a small monthly fee.

43. Answer: A

An incident report should be filled out immediately while details are still fresh in the therapist's mind.

44. Answer: A

As soon as the patient enters the clinic, the OT should begin to collect data based on informal observation. Posture, facial expression, and verbalizations are an integral part of the assessment. The medical history is informative but could bias the therapist about the client.

45. Answer: B

The dysphagia patient should never "wash down" food in the mouth. Food left in the mouth should be removed with a cloth or swab. All other precautions should be followed.

46. Answer: D

Speech is adequate but content is empty or vague. Dysarthria refers to difficulty in articulation. Pressured speech refers to rapid, hard-to-interrupt speech. Poverty of speech refers to limited amounts of speech that may be syllabic.

47. Answer: B

Impaired thought processes should alert the OT to the possibility of another disease.

48. Answer: A

Massage, elevation, gloves, and even dry cold packs will reduce edema, however, wet packs are contraindicated post surgery.

49. Answer: C

A narrow, shallow, and sturdy plastic- or rubber-coated spoon should be used to feed a child with reflex biting. The food will slide off easily on plastic. It is important to note that "plastic" does not mean disposable-type plastic ware typically served at parties. These might break with a strong bite.

50. Answer: C

Protocols differ from facility to facility. Some use 20% over resting heart rate as the stopping point of activity. Some use 120 beats per minute as the stopping rate. In either case the therapist could expect that the patient would have a pulse rate of at least 100 to 110 if engaged in strenuous exercise. Dyspnea, palpitations, and a glassy stare are all reasons to stop activity and notify the physician. The following are also signs to stop the activity and notify the physician: fatigue, faintness, dizziness, claudication pain in legs, excessive sweating, ataxic gait, irregular pulse, and high or low blood pressure.

Section Nine

1. Splinting of the wrist for the treatment of carpal tunnel syndrome should be static to prevent movement. At which position should the wrist be?
    A. 10 to 20 degrees extension
    B. 10 to 20 degrees flexion
    C. 5 degrees ulnarly deviated
    D. 30 degrees flexion

2. Prism glasses are ideal for:
    A. Patients with a halo or who are confined flat in bed
    B. Magnifying book pages
    C. Improving colors for low vision clients
    D. Not spilling drinks when patients have hand tremors

3. A child with spastic cerebral palsy has scissor gait. This means the hip muscles are:
    A. In flexion
    B. In abduction
    C. Internally rotated
    D. Externally rotated

4. Caffeine withdrawal includes all of the following *except*:
    A. Hallucinations
    B. Nervousness
    C. Insomnia
    D. Headache

5. An OT is leading a coping skills group for people with AIDS. Which of the following is inappropriate for the OT to tell clients during the group?
    A. Feeling guilt is common
    B. Homosexuals should not come out to their families at this time
    C. Discussion of terminal care
    D. Practice of safe sex is necessary

6. You are doing tactile stimulation with a group of three children. The children are lying on a mat and you are rolling a large ball over them. They like the feeling and ask you to do it again. What is the *best* response to the request?
    A. Say no, explain that they have had enough
    B. Repeat the activity, this time putting more pressure on the ball
    C. Say it's time to try something new
    D. Try bouncing the ball over them

7. Which of the following is *not* true about anorexia nervosa?
    A. The essential feature is binge eating
    B. Patients have a tendency toward perfectionism
    C. Body image is distorted
    D. Starvation and suicide are common causes of death

8. During an assessment of a client's occupational performance in the area of leisure, it is observed that the client chooses passive activities such as watching television and movie videos. The occupational therapist is assessing the client's motivation or:

    A. Volition

    B. Performance

    C. Competence

    D. Skills

9. An occupational therapist accompanies a client to the supermarket. The activity of supermarket shopping is an example of:

    A. Occupational context

    B. Occupational orchestration

    C. Occupational performance

    D. Occupational science

10. An occupational therapist facilitates a group activity every Friday for clients with mental illness within a social rehabilitation context. The specific question posed to this group is: "What are appropriate activities that you could participate in this weekend?" What type of group is the OT conducting?

    A. Peer support group

    B. Consultation group

    C. Developmental group

    D. Focus group

11. An occupational therapist is conducting a role play activity to modify the client's behavior. The goal of the intervention is to teach the client how to act in a classroom setting when he is confused and needs clarification of a topic. On what environmental aspect of the performance context is the occupational therapist focusing?

    A. Physical

    B. Social

    C. Temporal

    D. Cultural

12. All of the following conditions may lead to child abuse and neglect *except:*

    A. Low self-esteem of the parent(s)

    B. Mothers in their 20s

    C. Frustration with the child's toilet training

    D. Lack of support for family

13. Which of the following statements is *not* true regarding HIV and AIDS?

    A. Most infections secondary to HIV involve the central nervous system

    B. Prozac may be prescribed to deal with depression secondary to HIV

    C. No person should be given an HIV test without prior consent or knowledge

    D. HIV is a DNA retrovirus

14. Your patient is a young child with significant hearing loss due to a lesion in the middle ear. Which of the following areas might be a strength?

    A. Bilateral coordination

    B. Visual concentration

    C. Self-perception

    D. Play skills

15. In high velocity head injuries, a cranial nerve is commonly damaged. The results are a decrease in the sense of smell and, therefore, a decrease in appetite. What cranial nerve is this?

   A. I

   B. III

   C. IV

   D. V

16. A bowel program for the patient with a spinal cord injury includes all of the following *except:*

   A. Timing and a regular schedule

   B. Hot oral intake

   C. Suppository or digital stimulation

   D. Convenient time in the patient's schedule

17. In order to achieve the mechanical advantage of a stand pivot transfer, the client must *first*:

   A. Unlock the wheelchair

   B. Angle the wheelchair 90 degrees to the transfer location

   C. Scoot forward in the chair

   D. Do nothing, but the person providing the transfer must stand in front of the client with feet 30 cm apart

18. When comparing developmental norms between children with sight and children without sight, which is true concerning motor development?

   A. There is no difference

   B. Children who are blind develop more rapidly

   C. Children who are blind have motor delays

   D. Children who have sight have motor delays

19. Which of the following statements is *not* true concerning patients with chronic pain?

   A. Depression is frequent

   B. ADL activities may be avoided by the patient

   C. Pain is real to the patient

   D. Job performance is maintained

20. Which of the following goals would address poor coordination and atypical postures in a child with failure to thrive?

   A. Develop play skills

   B. Increase response to stimuli to normal range

   C. Increase gross motor to normal range

   D. Increase independence in ADLs

21. Factors used to indicate the severity of head injury and estimate the outcome include all of the following *except:*

   A. Glasgow Coma Scale

   B. Post-traumatic amnesia

   C. Galveston Orientation and Amnesia Test

   D. Assessment of tone and posturing using MMT

22. Which of the following goals is *most* meaningful and reflective of occupational performance?

   A. Client will learn five new coping strategies in group

   B. Client will decrease self-abuse by 50%

   C. Client will modify and improve anger management

   D. Client will improve physical self-concept by taking a daily shower

23. Effective treatment intervention does *not* include:
    A. Focusing on the occupational therapist's goals
    B. Identifying the client's baseline performance
    C. Writing measurable goals tied to occupational performance
    D. Exploring the client's needs, wants, and goals

24. An occupational therapist takes a group of three adolescent females to the nearby shopping mall. They were recently discharged from a residential facility and now live in a supervised apartment. This treatment intervention is known as:
    A. Home visits
    B. Environmental modification
    C. Community re-entry
    D. Activities of daily living

25. The occupational therapist designs a 10-step plan for brushing teeth. Positive reinforcement is identified for shaping the client's behavior along with appropriate prompts or cues. This type of treatment intervention is called:
    A. Functional skill training
    B. Reality orientation program
    C. Task adaptation
    D. Cognitive restructuring

26. The general rule regarding a person using alcohol after a severe head injury is:
    A. 4 to 6 weeks post injury
    B. Limit of one drink per day
    C. 2 years post injury
    D. Never drink again

27. The *most* common complaint of the patient with a spinal cord injury is:
    A. Depression
    B. Spasticity
    C. Fatigue
    D. Bladder control

28. Medications to reduce seizures in patients with head injuries might produce what side effect?
    A. Increase in emotional depression
    B. Increase in agitation
    C. Decrease in speech due to dry mouth
    D. Decrease in cognitive performance

29. Which of the following terms *best* describes a child who may incur developmental delays, disorders, or deficits because of factors occurring before, during, or after birth?
    A. Mental retardation
    B. High risk infant
    C. Failure to thrive
    D. Learning disabilities

30. Which of the following is *not* characteristic of normal adolescence?
    A. Acting out behavior
    B. Occasional delinquent acts
    C. Episodes of depression
    D. Increased closeness to siblings and parents

31. According to Anne Mosey, what term describes social structure, values, norms, and expectations shared by people?
    A. Human environment
    B. Social environment
    C. Non-human environment
    D. Cultural environment

32. Who among the following is *not* responsible for OT group treatment approaches?
    A. Gail Fidler
    B. Irvin Yalom
    C. Anne Mosey
    D. Mildred Ross

33. All of the following OT goals are appropriate to the motor component of a leather working task *except:*
    A. Increase bilateral coordination
    B. Increase eye-hand coordination
    C. Increase organization
    D. Increase hand strength

34. When taking patients with mental health disabilities outside, the OT needs to remember that patients on psychotropic medications:
    A. Sunburn easily
    B. Are sensitive to light
    C. Need to drink a lot of water
    D. Get muscle cramps easily

Use the following information to answer questions 35 and 36: Heterotrophic ossification can be a common medical condition of patients in rehabilitation programs.

35. People with all of the following may experience heterotrophic ossification *except:*
    A. Head injury
    B. Spinal cord injury
    C. Burns
    D. Multiple sclerosis

36. The *most* common site of heterotrophic ossification is the:
    A. Elbow
    B. Finger
    C. Hip
    D. Ankle

37. Allen's Cognitive Levels (ACL) provide a therapist with information on what could be expected of a patient at different levels. What activity would be *best* for a person with an ACL score of 1?
    A. Community activities such as shopping for hair care products
    B. Task activities such as lacing a wallet
    C. ADL activities such as brushing his or her teeth
    D. A simple activity such as listening to music in his or her room

38. The leading cause of death for a person with a spinal cord injury is:
    A. Cardiovascular problems
    B. Respiratory problems
    C. Urinary tract infections
    D. Spasticity

39. Quality assurance is all of the following *except:*
    A. Supported by AOTA
    B. No longer optional in hospitals
    C. In constant development and continuous in monitoring
    D. Required even in public school systems

40. The lateral curvature of the spine is:
    A. Kyphosis
    B. Spina bifida
    C. Scoliosis
    D. Rickets

41. Sacs of fluid located in areas of friction, especially in joints, are called:
    A. Bursae
    B. Fascia
    C. Ligaments
    D. Tendons

42. Positioning of a patient who is bed bound for an extended time should include all of the following *except:*
    A. Knees lifted by a pillow while supine
    B. One pillow under head while supine
    C. Frequent position changes
    D. No pillow under head, but one under knees while supine

43. What assessment tool is explicitly client-centered?
    A. Analysis of a client's task performance such as the COTE
    B. Performance of simulated tasks such as the KELS
    C. Observation of cognitive functioning such as the ACL
    D. A semistructured interview such as the COPM

44. What intervention is an example of cognitive restructuring?
    A. Finishing a five-step task successfully
    B. Changing five negative self-statements into positive ones
    C. Designing cue cards that list each individual step to task completion
    D. Educating the client's caregiver about safety precautions

45. The major occupational role of preschool children is:
    A. Player
    B. Student
    C. Worker
    D. Partner

46. Early intervention services for children from birth to 3 years old can be remedial or preventive to children with disabilities. Which of the following is *not* true about this approach?
    A. Play activities activate neurons
    B. Critical periods for brain development extend from early childhood to middle childhood
    C. The brains of young children are known to be highly plastic
    D. Cognitive, language, motor, perceptual, and emotional development are interdependent

Use the following information to answer questions 47 and 48: A 65-year-old widowed woman you are treating for an acute exacerbation of arthritis has been hinting around that she is having problems at home. Sensing that she does not want to talk about her problems in an open area, you ask her to meet with you in your office so you can have a private moment to speak with her. She tells you that she is "uncomfortable having sex with her new boyfriend." After talking further with her, she has identified joint pain as the problem.

47. Which of the following is crucial to the OT's ability to provide effective sexual counseling to this client or any other?
    A. Extensive awareness of anatomy and physiology
    B. Awareness of personal attitudes about sexuality, sex roles, and sexual preferences
    C. Details about the client's sexual history
    D. The referral process to a sex therapist

48. What is the *best* advice to give to this client at this time?
    A. The client should ask the boyfriend to give up sex until she is in remission
    B. Educate and encourage the client to try different sexual positions to reduce joint pain
    C. Suggest the couple try other romantic activities instead of sex until she feels better
    D. Tell the client that she should slow down and act her age

49. Which of the following is false regarding sensory stimulation for children with mental retardation?
    A. Helps to increase level of arousal
    B. Increases ability to focus attention
    C. Eliminates stereotyped behaviors
    D. Finding appropriate level of stimulation is important to success

50. A child has usually established hand preference by what age?
    A. 2
    B. 5
    C. 7
    D. 9

Section Nine Answers and Explanations

1. Answer: A

Flexion causes pain for the person with carpal tunnel syndrome, therefore 10 to 20 degrees extension is the correct position.

2. Answer: A

Prism glasses are eyeglasses that bend light 90 degrees so that a person lying on his or her back can watch television or read a book on his or her lap. B, C, and D are not true.

3. Answer: C

Scissor gait means that the hip muscles are internally rotated, in extension, and adducted.

4. Answer: A

Hallucinations do not occur. Nervousness, insomnia, and headaches do occur, with headaches as the most common.

5. Answer: B

Mental health treatment involves helping clients to self-disclose to family and significant others when they are ready. Helping the person deal with possible issues of rejection, guilt, shame, or anger are also roles of the occupational therapist.

6. Answer: B

Repeating the activity with more pressure allows for gradual gradation of proprioceptive input and allows the children to control the activity. Bouncing the ball over the children is both unsafe and frightening.

7. Answer: A

Binge eating is an essential feature of bulimia. B, C, and D are true.

8. Answer: A

A person's volition includes his or her free will, or ability to choose and make a decision. Within the model of human occupation, one's values, interests, and personal causation influence the volitional subsystem. Competence is the ability to meet the demands of one's environment. Performance is a collective outcome of many factors, such as physical and psychological areas, and includes one's skills, or proficiency, in a particular area of functioning.

9. Answer: C

Occupational performance is the act of doing occupation. Context refers to environments that are cultural, social, or physical in nature. Occupational orchestration refers to the qualities of occupation that include ideation, composition, execution, and ordering. Occupational science is a theory that studies form, function, and meaning of occupations.

10. Answer: D

Focus groups are organized around a specific theme and set of questions that are used to involve the members in a discussion of similar concerns. A peer support group is designed for persons with common conditions. A consultation group is a form of supervision that is offered by a practitioner to other clinical staff for professional development. The developmental group is Mosey's model that focuses on group interaction skills in progressive stages.

11. Answer: B

The social context refers to expectations that pertain to social interaction with others and role performance. The physical context refers to the specific non-human elements, such as the size of the room, colors of the walls, furniture, etc. Temporal aspects are separate from environmental aspects and refer to location of occupational performance in time, such as the client's age, developmental stage, etc. Cultural context refers to the customs, beliefs, and norms adapted by a particular group of people.

12. Answer: B

Children of teenagers are more likely to suffer from various problems, including abuse, neglect, inadequate health, hygiene, and nutrition. A, C, and D are true.

13. Answer: D

HIV is a RNA retrovirus that is primarily present in blood, semen, and cervical and vaginal secretions. To a small degree, it is also found in tears, breast milk, and cerebrospinal fluid of infected people.

14. Answer: B

Visual concentration and ability to refocus may become enhanced in children with hearing loss because of dependence on visual input. Bilateral coordination, self-perception, and play skills may be problem areas.

15. Answer: A

The olfactory nerve is commonly involved in high velocity head injuries.

16. Answer: D

Timing, hot oral intake, and suppositories or digital stimulation are all important factors of bowel programs. Consistency in a daily schedule allows the bowel to adjust to a predictable routine.

17. Answer: C

The patient must move forward in the chair to have his center of gravity over his feet when he comes to standing.

18. Answer: C

Delays are often present due to not using hands, fear of movement, and lack of visual stimulation.

19. Answer: D

Productivity and job performance are often interrupted due to chronic pain.

20. Answer: C

The problems stated are motor functioning, so the goal of increasing gross motor functioning to normal range is most appropriate. A, B, and D are possible goals for other problem areas.

21. Answer: D

MMT is a motor exam; all the others predict outcome to some degree.

22. Answer: D

Treatment goals should be stated in positive terms, be measurable, specific, and related to occupational performance. Answers A, B, and C do not reflect how the behavior is connected to a functional activity.

23. Answer: A

Effective treatment intervention is least concerned with the priorities of the occupational therapist and should remain centered on the client. Establishing the client's baseline performance is helpful because it allows both the client and practitioner to assess one's functioning level prior to intervention.

24. Answer: C

The purpose of a community re-entry group is to assist persons to establish occupational functioning in the designated environmental context.

25. Answer: A

This intervention involves the learning of a specific task through repetition and behavioral techniques. It is an effective technique for persons with cognitive deficits in the areas of self-care and work performance. Reality orientation programs assist persons who are confused to person, place, and/or time. Task adaptation is a concept used to modify and grade activities as needed. Cognitive restructuring is a complex intervention where distorted and/or negative thinking is replaced with positive and adaptive thoughts.

26. Answer: C

The outcome of therapy, as well as the long-term cognitive ability, demands at least 2 years avoidance of alcohol. Not drinking again is preferred.

27. Answer: C

Fatigue is the biggest long-term, chronic problem. Physical and mental energy requirements are high. A, B, and D can be controlled with medication or routine procedures.

28. Answer: D

The prophylactic use of anti-seizure medication can affect the patient's work in rehabilitation if there is a decrease in cognitive functioning caused by the medication.

29. Answer: B

High risk infant is a term used to describe a child with body system involvement, including respiratory, cardiovascular, metabolic, nutritional, immunologic, or ophthalmologic. Mental retardation is significant subaverage intellectual functioning and deficits in adaptive behavior. Failure to thrive is a disorder in which children fail to grow at a normal rate for their age, gender, or race. Learning disabilities are deficits in attention, memory, reasoning, or the ability to produce responses with desired and skilled behavior.

30. Answer: D

A normal developmental behavior for teenagers is the interest in developing peer relationships.

31. Answer: D

Social structure, values, norms, and expectations all describe cultural environment. Human environment describes individuals and groups of people. Social environment describes people with a social matrix of relationships. Non-human environment describes conditions, things, and ideas.

32. Answer: B

Yalom is traditional psychotherapy that occupational therapists have integrated into group treatment. Fidler developed the task-oriented group. Mosey coined the developmental OT group. Ross developed the integrated five-stage group.

33. Answer: C

Increased organization is a cognitive goal.

34. Answer: A

Some psychotropic medications leave the patient sensitive to sunburn. The OT must remind the patient to use sunscreen and protective clothing. B, C, and D might be due to other medications; the OT must be sensitive to all patient feedback.

35. Answer: D

People with MS tend to be more mobile and therefore less likely to develop heterotrophic ossification from prolonged immobility.

36. Answer: C

The hip is the most likely involved area with the elbow second. Shoulders and fingers can be involved but less than hips and elbows. Some textbooks say that the shoulder is most common, but recent research says hips and elbows are the focus.

37. Answer: D

A patient at ACL level 1 is unable to attend to his or her basic survival needs and, therefore, all the activities except listening to music would be too difficult.

38. Answer: A

People with spinal cord injuries are on par with society as cardiovascular problems are the leading cause of death for all people. B, C, and D are common problems for people with spinal cord injuries but manageable with medication.

39. Answer: D

Quality assurance (QA) is a required component to all hospital or rehabilitation programs that wish to have accreditation of third party reimbursement. In addition, QA is supported by AOTA as an essential component of practice. QA is constantly being developed and requires continuous monitoring. Public schools do not require QA; however, other systems of review are similar to QA in goals and methods.

40. Answer: C

Scoliosis is a lateral curvature of the spine. Kyphosis is a posterior curvature of the spine. Spina bifida is a congenital birth defect in which the spinal column does not close. Rickets is a skeletal condition due to the lack of vitamin D, usually seen in children.

41. Answer: A

Sacs of fluid near joint areas are called bursae. Fascia, ligaments, and tendons are also near joints but lack fluid.

42. Answer: D

While lying supine in bed, a pillow under the head and knees will reduce neck and back strain. Sidelying patients should bend their knees and use a pillow to support the head. Watch for hip contractures if the patient is bedridden for long periods.

43. Answer: D

A semistructured interview such as the COPM is created to measure the client's perception of his or her occupational performance over time. It is an example of a self-report evaluation rather than the occupational therapist's assessment of performance.

44. Answer: B

Cognitive restructuring involves the substitution of positive and adaptive thinking for self-defeating and maladaptive thinking. It is a technique that is used in the cognitive behavioral frame of reference. Answer B is one example of how to change a client's thoughts into a positive reframe. Answers A and C demonstrate cognitive skill development. Answer D is an example of a psychoeducational intervention that is useful for persons who have cognitive deficits.

45. Answer: A

The major occupation of this developmental stage is play during which children interact with others and learn about themselves as well as social expectations. Functioning as a student is the major role in middle childhood and adolescence. The roles of worker and partner are both major aspects of adulthood.

46. Answer: B

Critical periods for brain development extend from pregnancy to early childhood, when rapid growth and development occurs.

47. Answer: B

Sexual counseling is a component of occupational therapy. Competency and success is based on the OT's personal awareness, basic knowledge, and interpersonal skills. The OT needs to feel comfortable communicating with patients about their sexual issues and therefore must be comfortable with his or her own sexuality.

48. Answer: B

Sexual positions are helpful in relieving stress on joints. A, C, and D would be ineffective in addressing the issue.

49. Answer: C

While some evidence suggests that stereotyped behaviors may be lessened or interrupted, there is no evidence to show sensory stimulation can eliminate the underlying cause of behavior.

50. Answer: B

Hand preference is usually established by school age.

Chapter Six

Domain-Style Study Questions with Answers

Section One Domain-Style Questions

1. Mrs. Z is a 79-year-old widow who fell while carrying a bag of groceries up the few steps to her home. She fractured the neck of her right femur. While recovering in the hospital, she expresses her fear of going home alone. Select the *first* priority in the treatment considerations listed below.

    A. Provide a long-handled reacher, long shoe horn, and provide a review of precautions

    B. Practice bedside UE and LE dressing techniques

    C. Practice dynamic balance as the client comes to standing from bed or wheelchair

    D. A home visit to establish safety issues, recommendations for large equipment, and problem solving with the patient prior to discharge from the hospital

Use the following information to answer questions 2 and 3: As a result of a diving accident, Tom has damaged his spinal cord at the C-6 level. He is a complete tetraplegic.

2. Following 3 months of hospitalization and rehabilitation, he states to his therapist his most important goal is to be able to drive. His friends and girlfriend all live 100 miles from his hometown. He expects that he will live with his parents at least immediately postdischarge, and outpatient therapy will be in his hometown. Is driving a reasonable goal for Tom at this time?

    A. No. It must be a long-term goal. The patient needs to achieve independence in dressing, bathing, and transfers as a priority to the goal of driving

    B. Yes. The client's goals must be respected and the therapist may empower the client to direct his own care and thus feel in control of his environment

    C. No. The client would not have sufficient strength to drive

    D. Yes. Tom has the potential to drive; however, the cost would be prohibitive. The goal of driving should be delayed for at least a year or 2

3. Tom is very concerned about his ability to experience a full sexually expressive life following his injury. The treating therapist with basic understanding of SCI can address the client's sexual issues and provide intervention at a level that is clinically appropriate. The *best* choice of treatment for this client would be:

    A. The client is instructed in general bed mobility in order to reassure the client of his ability in this area

    B. The client is referred to a psychologist to address psychosocial sexual expression needs, and counseling can be provided as is indicated

    C. The client is asked to refrain from inappropriate discussion of sexual issues during the priority training of UE function

    D. The IADL goals of the client regarding sexual expression are addressed by utilization of the PLISSIT model

4. A computer operator is required to change how she performs her job in order to decrease the pain and other symptoms that impede her work performance and overall comfort in the work setting. The changes the client is required to make will also prevent a more chronic, painful situation from developing. An important quality the client requires to make an effective change is self-efficacy. What is self-efficacy?

    A. Self-efficacy is linked to self-esteem and overall view of an individual's body image

    B. Self-efficacy is a positive manifestation of self-confidence

    C. Self-efficacy is not likely to impact on the client's ability to make changes within her job setting

    D. Self-efficacy is the client's perception of the capacity to make successful change in performance

5. At the end of a group in the arts and crafts room of a locked psychiatric hospital, the OT finds a pair of scissors missing. The *first* thing the OT should do is:

    A. Walk around the room to see if the scissors are viewable

    B. Walk around the room and ask everyone if they have the scissors

    C. Stand by the door and ask everyone if they have the scissors

    D. Initiate the dangerous instrument search procedure

6. In a home care environment, 3 months post right CVA, the client's significant visual scanning problems require the therapist to focus on what *best* practice listed below?

    A. Motor learning

    B. Restoring the client's ability to scan the environment

    C. Modify the environment, have all like objects stored in one location

    D. Ask the caregivers to provide for the client's needs, anticipating her visual deficits

7. Harry is a 65-year-old male with diabetes and secondary peripheral vascular disease that resulted in a right lower extremity, above knee amputation. He does have a history of cardiac complication. He lives with his wife of 40 years and worries about his ability to attend to social and community activities. He is a VFW member and officer in the organization, serving on the honor guard. An important biomechanical frame of reference focus in treatment will be:

    A. Body image changes and the resultant issue of self-esteem and self-efficacy concerns for this client's adjustment to his amputation

    B. Strengthening of the UE and LE musculature primarily through the practice of functional tasks, such as dressing, bathing, and light exercise

    C. Dynamic balance component that requires subtle shifts in the center of gravity (COG), especially when coming to standing from the wheelchair; helping the client to adjust to changes with and without a prosthetic limb

    D. Educating the client as to stump care, which will include skin integrity inspection and donning and doffing his prosthetic leg

8. A client with systemic lupus erythematosus (SLE) has been on a high-dose oral corticosteroid for some time. Lately she has been complaining of increased fatigue when climbing steps and pain at rest in the right hip. What might your hypothesis be regarding these symptoms?

    A. The client could have an infection, although no fever was reported. The therapist could ask the patient to call her doctor

    B. The client could have myopathy of the proximal muscles of the lower extremity secondary to the corticosteroid

    C. The client has likely been overdoing her exercises and is fatigued, thus should take more rest periods, especially because of the corticosteroids

    D. The client is not reporting symptoms fully. The therapist could ask family members what symptoms or client behavior changes they have noted

9. Mary enters the clinic for her first visit to the pain management clinic. The symptoms listed below are exhibited by Mary spontaneously during your interview, and your hypothesis is overt pain behaviors. Select the behavior that confirms the hypothesis.

    A. Guarding, bracing, rubbing of the back with grimacing, and sighing during the interview

    B. Laughing and loud verbal response to your interview questions

    C. Sad demeanor, quiet response to questions with poor posture and unkempt appearance

    D. Client appears cheerful and eager to begin treatment with clearly defined goals and positive expectations for treatment

10. A female patient is admitted to an inpatient psychiatric facility for a 3-day evaluation after police were called to her home on a domestic disturbance call. When the police arrived, the couple was involved in a physical and verbal fight. The husband was intoxicated and was sent for a 3-day evaluation to another facility. The first 2 days, the female patient was going to leave her husband, but she is now crying and saying how much she misses her "love." What should the OT do?

    A. Model separateness and encourage the patient to develop boundaries

    B. Educate the patient to domestic violence

    C. Inform the patient that this new behavior is not healthy

    D. Ignore the negative behavior and focus attention elsewhere

11. An elderly, diabetic client with limited mobility is visited in the home by an OT. The apartment was very hot and the OT suspected that the client is dehydrated. The signs of dehydration are:

    A. No visible signs are present of dehydration

    B. Headache, confusion, dizziness when standing, and the skin feels clammy

    C. Decrease in body core temperature, dry skin, increased salivary function, and vomiting can be present

    D. Increased blood pressure, complaints of weight gain, no real observable motoric deficits, and client does have intact cognitive function

12. A client with a history of cardiac disease experienced a myocardial infarction (MI) 6 weeks ago. At present his tolerance for physical activity allows him to walk 2 miles per day with no ill effect. During his outpatient rehabilitation session, he mentioned to his therapist his fear of sexual activity. He fears death or injury to the heart during strenuous sexual activity. Can you reassure the client his stamina is adequate in terms of MET levels for sexual expression?

    A. No. You can only refer him to his physician

    B. No. You are not sure, so you tell him to refrain from sexual activity until you review reference materials

    C. Yes. A brisk walk or climbing a flight of stairs is equivalent to the MET level of sexual activity

    D. Yes. You know it is relaxing for the client to participate in sexual expression, and you doubt it could be a problem

13. For a client in the early phase of rehabilitation for treatment of acute inflammatory demyelinating polyradiculoneuropathy (Guillian-Barré syndrome), the *least* beneficial treatment would be:

    A. Gentle stretching of those joints that exhibit decreased PROM

    B. Active assistive exercise

    C. Daily ADL activities to the client's capacity

    D. Aggressive stretching to increase PROM

14. The OT creates a pamphlet for students in the physical education class of a junior high school. It emphasizes scoliosis as a disorder common in young girls and describes screening protocols within the school system. An exercise/support group the OT could recommend to the affected young women would be:
    A. Bike riding and/or walking 2 miles per day
    B. A yoga class with gentle stretching
    C. A strengthening group program with a focus on trunk extensors, abdominals, and hip extensor musculature
    D. A program that emphasizes trunk symmetry, balance reactions, and posture in general

15. The OT in a community mental health program based on the Fountain House model has been approached by the consumers to lead a group on alternative treatment techniques. The OT has only a basic understanding of alternative treatments. What is the *best* response?
    A. The OT should discourage the idea because of the possible conflicts with the consumers' current treatment
    B. The OT should acknowledge the request but ask for time to research the topics
    C. The OT should tell the consumers that she has no information or training in this area, and refer the consumers to an alternative treatment specialist
    D. The OT should tell the consumers that she has no information or training in this area, and refer the consumers to their medical doctor

16. The population of people over the age of 70 are at a high risk for burn injury. Prevention of accidents is essential. What would the focus of education and prevention in the well elderly be for burns?
    A. Educate the clients in the community with an overview of the problems in burn treatment and emphasize the cost of rehabilitation
    B. Education of agencies, particularly the VNA, to encourage referrals to OT when the issue of safety in home management is a concern
    C. Work on safety awareness in the acute care centers with all clients who have CVA
    D. Not much can be done in this area, the problem is too big and too costly

17. What type of visual supports are *most* effective for children with autism in the early stages of reading skills?
    A. Cue cards with objects and words
    B. Calendars and mini calendars
    C. Checklists
    D. Semantic maps

18. A mother complains that her 11-year-old son "can't find his way out of the bathroom" and is worried he will become hopelessly lost when he goes to a new middle school next academic year. The OT evaluates the student for directional dysfunction and agrees with the mother that there is a problem. The OT knows that rules at the middle school are tight to provide structure for the preteens, and lateness to class is not tolerated. The student is insisting that no one is to know he has a problem. His mother is supportive of this decision because she understands the peer pressure in middle school. The family has agreed to follow the OT's recommendations and practice skills over the summer. The OT has graded a list of activities that increases the level of directional skill. What is the *highest* level of directional skill?
    A. Body awareness
    B. Self as a reference point
    C. Environment as a reference point
    D. Others as a reference point

19. The greatest risk for an acute phase burn client is:
    A. Decreased ROM
    B. Decreased muscle strength
    C. Fear of disfigurement and thus depression
    D. Infection

20. An elderly woman, recently admitted to a nursing home, has become depressed and is refusing to leave her room. She is eating only minimal food. Her family and doctor have agreed to begin antidepressive medication. The nursing staff has referred the resident to OT for evaluation and treatment. The COPM was used for the evaluation, but the OT feels the client is too depressed and not accurately reporting her issues. What should the OT do *next?*

    A. Wait the 10 days that typically are needed for the resident to feel the effects of the medication, then give the COPM again

    B. Ask the nursing staff to get the patient out of bed and in a wheelchair. Take the resident on a tour of the OT department

    C. Make a short appointment with the resident during lunch and sit and talk with her

    D. Bring an animal-assisted therapy pet to her room and offer to let her pet it

21. The client is brought to the clinic by her husband, who appears very involved with his wife's illness. Sally has multiple complaints of chronic pain and does have LE edema, redness, and some soft tissue pain that warrants attention. Yet, she does miss appointments and generally appears to be noncompliant to the home program of exercises you prescribed. You may suspect:

    A. Your program has not found the "right" motivating plan to increase client compliance

    B. The client is a malingerer, not really willing to participate in therapy

    C. The client may be in an abusive relationship and domestic violence is the issue at the core of the non-compliance

    D. The client has a chronic problem that may not benefit from intervention, and the client needs to learn how to cope with her disorder

22. A client with bilateral amputation of the lower extremities is wheelchair dependent for most mobility needs. While in his wheelchair, he attempted to pick up something he wanted from the floor in front of him and the chair and client fell forward. The cause of the fall was:

    A. He was not wearing a seat belt to restrict the movement in the wheelchair

    B. The design of the wheelchair, likely a standard type, was poor

    C. He was cognitively impaired and was unrealistic as to his motoric abilities while in the wheelchair

    D. The center of gravity of the client was forward beyond the base of support within the wheelchair

23. Cultural competence in community-based practice is indicated when the therapist uses culturally sensitive health care intervention strategies. Select the answer that reflects an awareness level of cultural issues with the phrasing of a question during an evaluation.

    A. "You said that you generally go out to eat, so I do not need to evaluate home management and cooking concerns during our evaluation."

    B. "The making of a simple sandwich allows me to understand your home management competency; could you show me how you do this?"

    C. "Are there foods that you cannot eat together or that you must include in your diet? I want to be sure to consider that during our home management assessment."

    D. "Can you prepare food for yourself? If you respond yes, I will continue with the evaluation."

24. A client referred to the OT complains of problems with walking in the mall, a visually busy environment. Stair climbing, transfers from stand to sit, bathtub, and chair to stand are also problematic. She does not complain of any visual problems. The physical therapist has done a lower extremity MMT and the client's strength is WNL. You suspect the problem could be:

    A. Visual disturbance

    B. Vestibular disorder

    C. Motivational problem

    D. Psychosocial problem

25. The parents of a 26-year-old male would like their son to move out on his own so that they can sell their home and move to their retirement home in another state. The parents are very concerned that their son has a supported home life with continued services in the community mental health program in which he is currently participating. The OT is asked to evaluate the client and make a recommendation. After using the KELS, ACL, and a home visit, it is clear the client does not have the skills to be independent in the community. The client wants his own apartment if he cannot live with his parents. What should the OT do *first*?

    A. Arrange a meeting with the parents and the client to discuss future plans
    B. Talk with the client about the evaluation findings and ask if a meeting can be set up with the parents
    C. Let the parents know the evaluation results, finding out their time line for selling the house, and begin ADL and IADL training
    D. Refer the client to a housing specialist who can arrange a supportive housing system

26. Martha, as a result of her mastectomy, is experiencing lymphedema in the right upper extremity. The *most* important treatment role of the OT will be:

    A. Teaching life-long precautions
    B. Exercises to increase PROM in the involved limb
    C. Retrograde massage to the RUE
    D. The use of a pump sleeve with equal pressure over the edematous limb

27. A client with a TBI and a Glasgow Coma Scale score of 14, indicating a non-coma status, appears to have third cranial nerve damage as noted in your observation of strabismus, diplopia, and ptosis. The area of the brain *most* likely damaged is:

    A. Parietal lobe
    B. Brainstem
    C. Frontal lobe
    D. No clear indicator present to determine area of damage

28. A school system with a team approach to managing issues of students is interested in adding occupational therapy to their feeding and eating program. What is the *first* priority for the new OT team member?

    A. Proper positioning and safety issues regarding eating
    B. Providing interventions to increase developmental self-feeding
    C. Providing oral-motor interventions
    D. Assessing oral-motor issues

29. In evaluating a senior citizen's ability to keep a driver's license, the OT is *first* concerned with:

    A. Visual skills
    B. Cognitive functioning
    C. Physical functioning
    D. Brake reaction time

30. A person with a 20-year history of schizophrenia has learned that there are numerous jobs for people with computer skills. She would like to learn word processing because she "used to be good at typing." What should the OT do *first*?

    A. Place her in front of a computer and give her basic, simple instructions. Observe how she handles the situation
    B. Talk to her about her lack of general job skills and inability to hold other more basic jobs in the past
    C. Talk to her about her past work experience and current motivations for a word processing job
    D. Set up an appointment with the client for a work evaluation and see how she does

31. A person with a complete spinal cord injury at the C-5 level will have a spastic/reflexive bowel and bladder. The indication for training and management of the bladder will be:
    A. A reflexive bladder is an indication that a formal schedule with a strict routine of care will allow the client to manage with an intermittent catheterization program (ICP) of voiding
    B. The Crede's maneuver of applying external pressure over the abdomen to empty the bladder can be his voiding method
    C. The client will be provided with an indwelling catheter to be used on a more permanent basis
    D. The client will have voluntary control of his bladder function at the C-5 level

32. Deep vein thrombosis (DVT) is a risk factor in spinal cord injury (SCI) and cerebral vascular disease. Which of the following choices *best* describes the signs, symptoms, and course of treatment for a 65-year-old female client with a recent CVA experiencing a DVT?
    A. There are no specific signs or symptoms of DVT; however, anti-embolic stockings can be prescribed as a prophylactic
    B. The client experienced edema in the lower extremity and was placed on bed rest
    C. The client experienced edema but was allowed to continue the normal therapy routine
    D. The therapist noticed symptoms of pain, edema, and discoloration in the lower extremity. The therapist continued working with the client, making a note in the chart about the lower extremity

33. A computer operator presents the following symptoms during a work site assessment: tingling sensation at the level of the wrist and fingers, pain on prolonged supination of the forearm, and pain at the shoulder and neck all on the right side of the body. You suspect a possible compression injury of the brachial plexus proximally and median nerve distally. Your treatment priority would be:
    A. Wrist cock-up splint and reminders to the client to take frequent breaks during the day
    B. Wrist cock-up splint and readjustment of her chair and position of the computer keyboard
    C. Teach the client gentle positioning exercises that will promote nerve gliding as compression of the brachial plexus is present
    D. Advise the client to consider a job change as her condition is not likely to improve given the severity of her symptoms

34. Which position allows for gravity-assisted movement for play in a toddler with developmental issues?
    A. Supine
    B. Prone
    C. Side lying
    D. Sitting

35. The OT and therapeutic recreator are taking a group of seniors from a long-term psychiatric unit on a short hike to a picnic area. All the participants have been medically cleared for this activity. Nursing has provided sunscreen, bug repellent, and hats for the hikers. What other issue is *most* important?
    A. Appropriate social behavior
    B. Long pants to avoid tick or bug bites
    C. Medication that is typically given during meals
    D. Hydration

36. The nursing department in a skilled nursing and rehabilitation facility is asking the OT to assist with residents' hand care in the long-term program. These residents are not eligible for reimbursed OT services and have little rehabilitation potential, but the nurses are reporting tight hands that make bathing difficult. What should the OT do?
    A. Recommend that nurses keep rolled up washcloths in the residents' hands
    B. Make or buy hand cones for all the residents
    C. Evaluate each resident's hands and recommend needed equipment without reimbursement
    D. Make verbal suggestions to the nursing department because the residents are not eligible for services

37. A company is considering hiring an OT to consult with the employees to reduce musculoskeletal disorders and work absences. All of the following could be used to promote the use of OT at the work site *except:*
    A. Bill for services under the medical insurance of employees
    B. Reduced worker's compensation costs to the employer
    C. Respond to an Occupational Safety and Health Administration (OSHA) citation
    D. Respond to OSHA proposed ergonomic standards

38. A schoolteacher and principal of a local junior high has a history of peripheral vascular disease. Her left upper extremity was amputated above the elbow. She is a determined individual and continues to perform most tasks independently, including sewing (she is an avid quilter). She has developed pain in the right shoulder due to a rotator cuff injury secondary to overuse. She is having repair surgery and is most anxious regarding her reduced capacity for function during the rehabilitation phase following her surgery. What approach to the client will be the *most* beneficial?
    A. COPM, client centered with the client directing the therapy focus
    B. Biomechanical—the issue is compensation for loss of function
    C. Rehabilitative—the client will need to relearn function following surgery and thus adapt to the change in functional status
    D. Psychosocial—the client is unable to admit limitations and persists in tasks that are counterproductive to maintaining remaining function

39. A 26-year-old medical student was recently diagnosed with multiple sclerosis. Her symptoms include visual difficulties, decreased strength in the lower extremity, fatigue, and visual disturbances. She states her primary goal is to attend her classes and be with her peers. The occupational therapist will *first* address:
    A. Encouraging the client to adapt goals for a more realistic long-term plan
    B. Encouraging the client to attend class from home via a distance learning program
    C. Starting a program of progressive exercises to increase endurance
    D. Energy conservation, safety, and balance exercises

40. During a team meeting, a client who keeps fainting is discussed. The client is on several psychiatric medications but evaluation of the medication has shown these are not the cause of the fainting. The client's vital signs are normal. Several staff feel the client is simply exaggerating lightheadedness to get staff's attention. The OT has noticed the fainting seems to happen more with activity than when staying still. The OT suspects possible:
    A. Blood pressure problems
    B. Anxiety and hyperventilation
    C. Migraines
    D. Vestibular disorder

41. A 65-year-old male with a fracture of the right femur, his second fracture in 1 year, is somewhat overweight at 290 pounds. He is a skilled craftsman, self-employed, strong willed, and independent in most areas of self-care. He contracted polio at age 1, and his doctor feels that he is experiencing a post-polio episode with decreased general strength and endurance. He has been utilizing loftstrand crutches for many years to ambulate with markedly reduced strength in the lower extremity. The client at this time is using a manual wheelchair, but his goal is to discontinue use of the wheelchair and hopes to be able to transfer independently in the home. The primary assessment that is required to develop a treatment plan for this client would be:
    A. ADL status, especially dressing skills
    B. Avocational interests and develop leisure time skills plan
    C. Safety in the home, especially with regard to transfers
    D. Sensory status and overall endurance

42. A client who uses a power wheelchair and has severe contractures is developing pressure sores despite earlier low technology interventions. The doctor has asked the OT for an opinion on a tilt or recline system to relieve the pressure. Which is likely the *most* effective?

    A. Tilt

    B. Recline

    C. Whichever would allow the client to transfer easiest

    D. Either one, consider cost and mobility first

43. An assisted living facility has expressed some interest in finding out more about occupational therapy. Currently, an OT from the local visiting nurse agency visits one of the residents for home therapy after a stroke. All of the following services are appropriate for the assisted living facility *except:*

    A. Consulting with residents through home evaluations on ways to reduce falls

    B. Consulting with administration on developing a social-emotional system that involves all residents

    C. Provide direct OT services billing through Medicare or Medicaid

    D. Educate family or home health aides on ways to better facilitate independence

44. The OT working for a large school system has been assigned the additional responsibility of being the ADA consultant for the employees with disabilities. What is the *first* step in managing this task?

    A. Subscribe and read journals related to ADA, workplace issues, and laws

    B. Call local human resources personnel and ask for copies of policies they use

    C. Attend training or conferences on ADA advocacy

    D. Obtain and read the ADA and administrative guidelines from the Equal Employment Opportunity Commission

45. A couple dealing with the early to middle stages of Alzheimer's disease has decided that the person with the disease will remain home as long as possible. The OT has recommended all of the following safety adjustments to the home *except:*

    A. Place a deadbolt on the front door

    B. Cover the cellar door with a sheet

    C. Remove the lock on the bathroom door

    D. Remove the stoppers on the sinks and tubs

46. An OT is working with an elderly man with peripheral visual field loss. As part of a grant from a local service club, the client is picked up at his home and transported to the outpatient clinic where the OT works. The client has reported satisfaction with his treatment, and the OT has arranged a home visit to evaluate the client's integration of learning to his context. During the home visit, his daughter reports how frustrated she is with her father knocking over cups of water during dinner when he reaches for other items. What should the OT do to address this issue?

    A. Have the client switch to a sports bottle-type cup for water

    B. Teach the client to visually scan in an organized manner to avoid overlooking items on the table

    C. Have the daughter switch to a tablecloth that contrasts with the cups so the client will see it better

    D. Ask the eye doctor to address the issue during his next visit

47. A one-handed high school freshman athlete is at risk of losing his athletic status because of low grades. His teachers report that the major issue is not his cognitive understanding but his unreadable and messy work. The OT reviews his record to see that he has been offered keyboarding techniques but prefers handwriting because of speed. The student says that his athletic status is most important to him and does not understand why the teachers are "picking on" his handwriting. The student is willing to reconsider keyboarding to meet his goal. What is *most* important in successful one-handed keyboarding?

    A. Training

    B. Positioning

    C. Adapted keyboard

    D. Data entry skills

48. A former client and his family have called your outpatient facility and reported that because of their satisfaction with services rendered when they were in rehabilitation, they would like to pay for consulting services as they get ready to build a new house. The client would like to have the new house built with environmental controls and electronic aids to improve his management of ADLs. The licensure laws in this state allow for services to be rendered without doctor's orders, and the facility is interested in exploring new non-medical services. The architect needs to know what type input the electronic devices will use. The client has UE movement and reports his most important goal is socializing. What inputs might be *first* evaluated?

    A. Switch

    B. Voice

    C. Serial, computer

    D. Combination

49. A parent reports frustration with the attempt to encourage her child to stand. She adds that the child cries in standing and gets things done faster if allowed to crawl. The parent knows standing is important to walking but cannot handle the crying. The OT recommends play activities during standing. What play activities during standing are *not* recommended?

    A. Singing and rocking side to side or front to back

    B. Bright socks and bells on the ankles

    C. Reaching for toys slightly out of reach

    D. Standing in front of a mirror

50. An OT with less than 1 year experience has joined an OT department with 11 other OTs and OTAs. The department manager wants to facilitate everyone's professional development, so he has randomly assigned each person a month where he or she will present a 45-minute inservice on topic of choice related to work. The new OT is assigned next month's inservice and does not want to do this because she is new. What should the managing OT do?

    A. Give the new OT a different month so she has more experience

    B. Have the new OT keep the inservice date. Encourage the new OT to present a new topic learned in school

    C. Excuse the new OT from the inservice since she is new to the job

    D. Have the new OT keep the inservice date and learn a topic in the next month

Section One Answers and Explanations

1. Answer: D

The transition to the home is most difficult and requires the most support for the patient. A home care therapist can be arranged for the client. Safety of the client is the primary issue in this case. The treatment considerations of A, B, and C are issues that should be addressed, however, studies indicate transfer of learning when practicing ADLs does not always carry over from the hospital to the home setting. The short stay in the hospital warrants the review of ADLs, equipment, and precautions within the OT clinic; however, the most significant results from long-term patient-independent function will be the practice of life skills in the home setting.

2. Answer: B

The client's goals must be respected. The goal of driving would result in working on many areas in order to achieve the main goal. Thus, UE strengthening exercises (answer B), wheelchair mobility, increasing endurance, problem solving, and planning ahead will all foster the motivation. Answer A is not a reasonable response in that a person with C-6 level function may not be able to achieve full independence in dressing, bathing, and transfers. In any event, the effort required would be exhausting and thus delay the patient's goal of driving. The patient does not express ADLs as a priority. This devalues the client's view of his own self-efficacy. A person with the functional ability at the C-6 level is able to drive a vehicle that has been properly outfitted with the necessary hand controls and extra equipment needed to drive safely (answer C). The cost of an adapted vehicle is high (answer D), although not prohibitive. The loss of patient confidence in his ability is not worth the price of delaying the early attempt to explore Tom's driving potential.

3. Answer: D

All therapists, no matter what their level of education on sexual rehabilitation issues, can provide patients the permission (P) to ask questions. Limited information (LI) can be provided in the way of printed material and then specific suggestions (SS) may be the level that requires more training on the part of the therapist. IT is the intensive therapy stage and this would be provided by a formally trained therapist/psychologist for those clients with premorbid history of dysfunction. This four-stage model respects the comfort and knowledge base of the client and the therapist. Answer A is a subset of areas that could be therapeutic but avoids the complexity of the need for more direct services regarding Tom's sexual expression. PLISSIT program does not require a referral to a psychologist as outlined in answer B. If the client elects to bring the concern to the clinical milieu, support can be provided by the treating therapist who then can determine the next step for the client and therapist. Answer C clearly gives the message that it is not okay to ask about his concerns or discuss his feelings. This response by the therapist could undermine the trust that needs to be nurtured in a therapeutic program for a person with a spinal cord injury.

4. Answer: D

Self-efficacy is essential for the positive belief that change of behavior is within a client's potential. A and B are sometimes linked to self-efficacy, but this is a concept very separate from body image or self-confidence. Answer C is not true.

5. Answer: C

If the clients were allowed in the arts and crafts room then they are likely to have behavior that immediately excuses initiating the dangerous sharps policy. The OT should, for safety's sake, position herself between the clients and the door and ask for the missing scissors. Likely, the sharps were simply misplaced and will be found immediately. If not, the OT should call for assistance.

6. Answer: C

If all the items needed for self-care are placed in one plastic container, the need to scan would be diminished. Answer A is vague and would not address the problem. Answer B is a time-consuming treatment that may or may not be successful. Time constraints warrant an immediate solution; however, answer D does not allow the patient any opportunity to accommodate to the loss via adaptation.

7. Answer: C

The issue of dynamic balance is essential for the patient to understand the safety considerations with shifts in COG. Furthermore, the client is most anxious regarding his ability to be out in the community. This will lead to a sense of control and self-efficacy, as he will be able to attend to VFW activities, and he will be more accepting of the total rehabilitation program.

8. Answer: B

Myopathy is a common side effect of corticosteroids secondary to the inhibition of protein synthesis. Corticosteroids do place a client at risk for infection and a host of other disorders affecting multiple systems. In answer A, indeed the client could be at risk for an infection, but there are no other signs like fever to support that view. Answers C and D do not directly address the problem of the client's condition.

9. Answer: A

These symptoms confirm overt pain behaviors and the conclusion of a behavioral response to pain. Answer B is not a clear predictor of overt pain behaviors. Answer C indicates possible depression and is unclear as to pain response. Clearly answer D does not indicate pain behaviors.

10. Answer: A

The OT should model separateness, healthy expression, and boundaries because the client is currently dealing with co-dependency issues and does not know how to behave as a separate individual in a relationship. Education about violence can be helpful only after a person sees the reality of the relationship. Ignoring the behavior can be appropriate in a behavioral conditioning frame of reference but not likely effective in short-term acute evaluation.

11. Answer: B

Other symptoms can be included, but those listed are most notable, and the heat of the apartment along with the secondary condition of diabetes makes dehydration likely. Answer A is not true. Answers C and D are the exact opposite of the signs of dehydration.

12. Answer: C

Answer A is poor in that it does not address the issue. Answer B does not deal with the matter in a timely fashion. Answer D does not use scientific data to justify the response.

13. Answer: D

Overstretching and overuse of painful muscles may result in a prolonged recovery period or a lack of recovery. All the other choices would be appropriate for this client.

14. Answer: C

This young age group within a school system would benefit from the peer support concept. The risk of osteoporosis is high in this population of young women with scoliosis; thus, a dietary element could also be introduced.

15. Answer: B

The OT should acknowledge her lack of current information but should seek information from both alternative medicine resources and opposing scientific sources. Some alternative treatments are helpful in conjunction with medical treatment and some simply have no scientific proof or are contraindicated. The informed consumer can make informed decisions.

16. Answer: B

Educate the VNA and perhaps the agency on aging to provide educational seminars and pamphlet production to encourage safe home management techniques in the clients they serve. All other answers limit effectiveness.

17. Answer: A

Cue cards with pictures and words help the student develop reading skills while also acting as visual reminders and reinforcing social skills. Cue cards without pictures are also helpful once the student begins reading. Calendars and semantic maps provide additional ways of organizing information once basic concepts are mastered.

18. Answer: D

Body awareness, self, environment, and others as reference are the development of directional skills. This student likely has body awareness and self as reference (intrapersonal space) mastered but needs to develop skills in extrapersonal space. Environment reference sees the body in relationship to objects in space. Others as a reference point understand that every person has a different perspective of direction than the child's perspective.

19. Answer: D

Infection is the single most serious concern during the acute phase of burn management. All the other choices would be a more serious issue in the emergent phase or rehabilitation phase of the client's overall recovery program.

20. Answer: D

The resident is sending a clear message that she does not want human contact. Despite knowing this is not healthy, relationships cannot be forced. A pet introduced to the resident (if she accepts) is the logical next activity to try. An animal-assisted trained dog might be brought to her bedside to see if she will pet it. A small lap pet, such as a bunny, might also be tried.

21. Answer: C

Studies indicate as high as 50% of female clients with chronic pain are in abusive relationships; thus, the OT needs to explore this issue with the client. The fact that her husband is always there indicates some issue of concern. All the other answers are less likely.

22. Answer: D

The biomechanical frame of reference would emphasize the issue of wheelchair use considering the center of gravity (COG) of the person within the chair. Consideration is also given to the COG of the wheelchair. Answer B starts to address the problem, as the client should not be in a standard chair. Answer A is unrealistic for an active wheelchair user. Answer C is unclear, as there is not an indication that cognitive dysfunction is present.

23. Answer: C

The therapist is clearly trying to establish the concerns of the client regarding cooking and food preferences. Answer A does not address the issue of whether the client can prepare food if required to, even though it respects the client's current situation. Answer B undermines the complexity of home management and would not result in realistic data on the client skill level. Answer D allows for avoidance of the complex issue of home management.

24. Answer: B

The client with a vestibular disorder has poor balance, vertigo, blurred vision, nausea, and spatial disorientation issues. There is little evidence to suggest any other answer.

25. Answer: B

The client is a legal adult, and the OT needs to have his permission to talk to the parent unless the parent maintains guardianship. Once permission is obtained, the issue of skills and resources can be addressed.

26. Answer: A

The risk of infection (sepsis) is great, thus education to prevent or maintain status is essential, especially skin care, no needle sticks to the involved limb, protect the hand at all times, and avoid tight clothing. Answer B can be important but active exercise is important too. Answer C, retrograde massage, does very little to resolve edema. Manual lymph drainage is a preferred treatment. Equal pressure pumps are not recommended.

27. Answer: B

The brainstem is a common head injury location and the cranial nerve involvement reinforces that hypothesis. Answers A and C would require more signs of dysfunction like arousal problems, speech, and/or language deficits. The choice of D is not indicated.

28. Answer: A

Safety is always first and positioning aids in feeding. All the other answers are appropriate for the OT to address, but safety is first.

29. Answer: B

All of the skills are important in driving, but cognitive skills can impact the other skills and affect the person's ability to make sound driving judgments.

30. Answer: C

The client is motivated to pursue this avenue and the OT does not want to negate this motivation even if the goal may be unrealistic. Begin with talking to the client to understand and support the motivation, follow up with a formal or observational evaluation if necessary.

31. Answer: A

A is the best answer and preferred choice, as the client's risk of infection is reduced. Answer B is used with a passive bladder or hyporeflexive bladder. Some clients at C-5 may require an indwelling catheter, but this is not the best choice. A patient with C-5 complete transection of the cord will not have voluntary bladder control.

32. Answer: B

The patient should be immobilized or on bed rest until the acute danger and episode has receded. The client would initially display signs of edema, pain, and skin discoloration. DVT is a very serious situation and does require immediate notification of the physician and medical team. Answer A is false; there are signs of DVT and tests to evaluate the presence. In answer C, the client should not be allowed to continue the therapy routine but instead be placed on bed rest as in B. The therapist in answer D made the wrong choice for the best care of the client.

33. Answer: C

The client's symptoms indicate compression of the brachial plexus. The proximal signs indicate more than carpal tunnel syndrome. Answers A and B are too simplistic, and answer D is too dramatic without true justification.

34. Answer: C

Side lying brings the child's arms and legs to midline and provides gravity assistance to movement for play. The child can see the hands and begins to coordinate movements. Pillows and rolled up towels can support the position. The other positions require more resistance to gravity and may also be appropriate for addressing developmental issues.

35. Answer: D

Hydration is especially important with seniors who may be on several medications and are always at risk of dehydration because of their age. The other issues are also important but can be addressed after hydration.

36. Answer: C

If the OT is employed by the facility, services can be provided without reimbursement issues. If the OT is employed by a contracted agency, the facility likely has an arrangement that allows long-term residents to have access to services. The OT has an ethical responsibility to ensure everyone has access to services. From a treatment perspective, answer A is rarely an acceptable plan. Soft washcloths only encourage flexion, making the problem worse. Hand cones or commercially available equipment that is shaped like a carrot is more appropriate. Nursing often uses washcloths and should be educated that this will make the hand tightness worse. The exception would include extremely fragile residents for whom quality of life is more important.

37. Answer: A

A company cannot bill their own ergonomics consultant under their own medical insurance. The company would have to pay for these services in some other way but would likely see reductions in medical and worker's compensation costs as employees reduced injuries related to work.

38. Answer: A

The client needs to feel in control; thus, reviewing with the client prior to surgery the potential areas of concern will be helpful. Problem solving for issues that will be present following the surgery during the rehabilitation phase will also be helpful for this client. Answers B and C do not consider the style the client has used to cope with for years. Without acknowledging the client's way of being, intervention will be frustrating for all involved. Answer D would be time consuming and, in this situation, not a focus for treatment. Answer A allows for the possibility of discussion of problem areas with the therapist.

39. Answer: D

The client's most important goal is to attend class. This primary goal then is the focus in treatment in client directed care. This young woman clearly has her goals prioritized and sees this as a motivational and stabilizing issue.

40. Answer: D

Since vital signs (blood pressure, pulse, and respiration) are fine, answers A and B are not likely. It is possible to have migraine symptoms without having the painful headache, but this is extremely rare and not likely to only produce fainting. Since fainting seems to be with movement, a vestibular disorder might be present and should be evaluated by an ear, nose, and throat doctor.

41. Answer: C

Home safety is most important, as this client may be unrealistic about his changes in overall status, including strength, endurance, and general mobility. The client is married, but the wife may not be able to provide assistance that would significantly change the outcome. Answers A, B, and D all have merit; however, in the priority the issue of mobility and safety are most important. The client needs assistance in learning to problem solve as new issues regarding ability are present. This patient is self-motivated to work hard to maintain independence but requires help in a realistic plan to cope with his present limitations.

42. Answer: A

Tilt and recline wheelchairs are used for a variety of issues including pressure relief, head and neck control, sleep, improved functional access, and regulating blood pressure. A tilt system does not change the angles of the body as does a recline system. The tilt is most appropriate for contractures that will not allow for changing body angles. Tilt and recline systems do add costs and weight to power chairs and this needs to be considered as well.

43. Answer: C

Assisted living centers promote independence. Although a person may be eligible for direct OT services through a third party payer, the focus in assisted living is prevention.

44. Answer: D

All the answers are good ways to become educated about ADA; however, the OT should first obtain the law and guidelines.

45. Answer: A

A deadbolt should not be placed on the front door because a person with Alzheimer's could lock out the spouse when he or she steps outside for the newspaper or mail. The bathroom door lock should be removed so that the patient does not lock out the spouse. The cellar door can be hidden with a sheet so the person does not try to open the door and gain access to dangerous supplies or tools. The stoppers should be removed to avoid flooding from forgetting to turn off the water. In addition, scatter rugs and stove knobs should be removed.

46. Answer: B

Adapted equipment is not considered until other issues are addressed. The issue is not just spilling water but overlooking items when looking for a different item. Changing the cup or tablecloth may be appropriate if the family does not mind the change, but many families have rituals at dinner and a sports bottle or contrasting tablecloth might not fit their context. The eye doctor might be appropriate if other issues are involved but not necessarily appropriate if cognitive training addresses the problem.

47. Answer: B

Position including the user's relationship of body to the keyboard, hand placement, size, and range of motion of the hand, size of fingers, and the relationship to the size of keys. Training and keyboard are addressed after position. In this specific class, the benefits in keyboarding will likely show immediate results in quality of academic work, allowing the student to maintain athletic status. The correct positioning will be least intrusive and likely not resisted by the teen. Positioning also reduces secondary disabilities like carpal tunnel syndrome, which could affect the athlete.

48. Answer: C

Computer electronic aids for daily living would be a logical first step because of the ability to increase socialization through chat rooms and email. Computers also provide the most variety for use over switches, which are on/off or voice and limited to vocal commands. Switches and voice may also be used in selected areas of the house for specific needs but computers allow greater socialization.

49. Answer: B

Bright socks or toys on feet will encourage the child to look down and make balance less successful. The other play activities encourage correct position and balance—the needed skills for walking.

50. Answer: B

The managing OT should encourage the new OT to present something she knows about that the more experienced OTs and OTAs may not have had in school. Changing the date involves another person and is not needed because the new OT has the skills necessary to perform the inservice. Mosey's principles of teaching and learning that are basic to patient education can also be used by the new OT herself in teaching and learning.

Section Two Domain-Style Questions

1. Children with attention deficit hyperactivity disorder (ADHD) may also have learning disabilities. What additional evaluation should the OT do when evaluating a child with ADHD?

    A. Occupational performance

    B. Activities of daily living

    C. Handwriting

    D. Memory

2. A client you are seeing for hand rehabilitation mentions that he also has gout and that "it is flaring up because of all the picnics he went to over the long 4th of July weekend." He adds that the doctor did not give him any new medication because of the NSAIDs he is taking for his hand. He asks the OT for recommendations. The OT recommends all of the following *except:*

    A. Reduce alcohol ingestion

    B. Consider a weight reduction program

    C. Restrict fluid intake to reduce swelling

    D. Keep the doctor updated on all other medications he is taking

3. A toddler with failure to thrive is referred for home evaluation and treatment for developmental issues. The toddler is below the fifth percentile for weight for her age. Her mother reports that every meal is a battle. The OT recommends all of the following *except:*

    A. Allow snacking and juice consumption throughout the day

    B. Incorporate play and playful interactions into meals

    C. Consider the child's emotional needs

    D. Consider age-appropriate portions of foods

4. A baby lying in supine is developing midline control, moving arms against gravity, and body awareness of the lower extremities. What activity is *least* appropriate to facilitate gravity-resisted play in supine?

    A. Put bracelets or rattles on the baby's ankle

    B. Have parents make faces and sounds to attract the baby's interest

    C. Use a mirror to encourage the baby to lift the head

    D. Hold toys at different positions

5. Marketing occupational therapy services includes all of the following *except:*

    A. Needs assessment

    B. Environmental assessment

    C. Organizational assessment

    D. Market analysis

6. A consulting classroom OT has been asked for recommendations to help a third-grader stay in his classroom seat, as he usually wiggles around until standing and then disrupts others. The student was getting services from special education, and his parents had him enrolled in a sensory integration program after school. What recommendation could result in improved focus on tasks?

    A. Replace the static classroom chair with an inflatable ball

    B. Evaluate for motor movement issues

    C. Replacing the classroom chair with a firm chair with side arms

    D. Using a lap tray on a soft chair to keep the student focused

7. A senior citizen is referred to a driver's evaluation program because his optometrist thought he was "a bit" confused during his last visit. He arrives at the clinic driving alone in his older-model car. What evaluation should the OT use *first*?

    A. An interview to establish the person's perception of skills

    B. A general cognitive and physical assessment of functioning

    C. Clinical evaluations such as the Trailmaking Test or the Short Blessed Exam

    D. Visual tests for acuity and peripheral vision

8. Changes in Medicare funding and insurance reimbursement have led to changes in the traditional roles of occupational therapists. The *most* effective way to advocate for legislation that supports the profession is forming a collaboration with:

    A. Lawyers

    B. Medical doctors

    C. Other rehabilitation specialists such as physical therapists

    D. Lobbyists

9. An OT has been asked to consult with the family of a 69-year-old woman recovering from a left cerebrovascular accident. The woman is medically stable and will be leaving the acute care hospital for a 1-week rehabilitation stay in a local nursing facility. The family's priority is home care rehabilitation as soon as possible. The OT must consider assessment of all of the following *except*:

    A. Environment

    B. Social support

    C. Financial support

    D. Medical status at admission

10. The OT in a small community program has been given permission to hire an OTA. During the interview process, the OT should ask the applicant all of following *except*:

    A. Semistructured, open questions asked of all applicants

    B. Personal characteristics

    C. Why he or she wants to leave his or her current job

    D. Job-related issues and characteristics

11. An OT is anticipating the opening of a new dementia unit in the skilled nursing home in which she works. The purpose of the unit is to provide assessment and referral for the appropriate level of care, from returning to independence to 24-hour nursing care. The OT wants to assess both performance areas and components as they relate to function. Which assessment would be *best*?

    A. Allen's Cognitive Levels

    B. Cognitive Performance Test

    C. Kohlman Evaluation of Living Skills

    D. Mini-Mental Status Exam

12. In what position should the neck be splinted for a pediatric patient with burns?

    A. 10 degrees hyperextension

    B. 10 degrees flexion

    C. Flexion, as much as possible

    D. 0 degrees, neutral

13. A hyperactive gag reflex may be normalized by:

    A. Icing the lips and having the patient say "Ooo"

    B. Offering resistance to opening the jaw

    C. Walking a tongue depressor toward the back of the tongue

    D. Sucking through a 6-inch straw and gradually increasing the straw length

14. If a patient slightly cuts his finger while cutting vegetables in the ADL kitchen, the OT should follow universal precautions and then:
    A. Call a medical emergency
    B. Hand the patient a gauze and ask him to apply pressure to the cut
    C. Call his nurse to the kitchen
    D. Call the OT supervisor for assistance

15. A patient with bilateral proximal UE weakness would benefit from what type of equipment while self-feeding?
    A. Enlarged handles on utensils
    B. Scoop dish
    C. Rocker knife
    D. Mobile arm supports

16. Dantrium (dantrolene) is often given to patients with spinal cord injuries to decrease spasticity. A side effect of this medication might include:
    A. Seizures
    B. Liver toxicity hepatitis
    C. Hallucinations
    D. Decreased blood pressure

17. Energy conservation techniques include all of the following *except:*
    A. Sit to work
    B. Limit amount of work
    C. Organize storage
    D. Plan one day at a time

18. An adolescent with a spinal cord injury is refusing to cooperate in the formal occupational therapy assessment at admission. What is the *best* option for the OT?
    A. Administer a different assessment
    B. Use informal methods at first
    C. Discontinue the assessment and wait until the patient is more cooperative
    D. Tell the teenager that you will have to tell his parents

19. Which of the following patients would *best* benefit from a wheelchair with removable arms?
    A. The head injured client who might get confused by arm rests
    B. The elderly patient with ataxia who needs to get to the tub or sink
    C. The patient with a T-4 spinal cord lesion who wants to use a transfer board
    D. The patient with Alzheimer's disease who cannot reach dropped items

20. A patient who does not speak your language is resistive and frightened to transfer from the bed to a wheelchair to go to therapy. What is the occupational therapist's *best* approach?
    A. Answer his "No, no" with a firm "Yes you can, I will help you"
    B. Ask the nursing aides to transfer the patient before you come up
    C. Demonstrate the transfer with another therapist
    D. Put a transfer belt on the patient and transfer him while making eye contact

21. A patient recovering from a mastectomy and undergoing chemotherapy will have many issues in occupational therapy, including both physical and psychosocial rehabilitation. All of the following are appropriate *except*:

    A. If the patient initiates the questions first, the therapist can answer questions about prognosis, treatments available for cancer, and pain medications

    B. Teach energy conservation and work simplification techniques

    C. Use counseling skills to address body issue and role changes

    D. Provide strengthening exercises and share MMT results with the patient

22. Quality assurance (QA) requires the development of indicators as variables that indicate quality care of the patient. All of the following would be appropriate occupational therapy indicators in a mental health service *except*:

    A. Occupational therapy assessment initiated within 24 hours of admission

    B. QA plan will be monitored monthly

    C. Patient involvement in goal setting is indicated by patient signature on the OT treatment plan

    D. Patient verbally reported feedback during treatment as documented in the progress notes

23. During an occupational therapy session, a male client begins to hyperventilate as he discusses his fears and anxieties. The occupational therapist calmly asks him to focus on her face as she begins to give directions for a deep breathing exercise. The purpose of this activity is:

    A. To cure the client

    B. To divert the client's attention from his anxiety

    C. To allow the occupational therapist to gain external control

    D. To encourage the client to tolerate the session

24. A newly admitted client is asked to complete an activity schedule designed to show how she balances self-care, work, and leisure. What is the activity goal for this session?

    A. To create self-concept

    B. To assess time management

    C. To restore self-expression

    D. To modify self-control

25. A client was admitted to a psychiatric unit and treated for depression. The occupational therapist gives the client an interest checklist and asks about activities that this client enjoyed in the past. This information will be useful in determining what aspect of occupational treatment implementation?

    A. To elevate mood

    B. To restore leisure pursuits

    C. To improve depression

    D. To minimize sadness

26. What activity would *best* allow an occupational therapist to observe a client's level of competence in the performance area of work/productive activity?

    A. Completing a 200-word puzzle in the hospital day room

    B. Cleaning up the activity room following a craft group

    C. Preparing a family meal in the client's kitchen at home

    D. Exercising at the local gym

27. Which of the following activities is *best* suited to assess a female client's cultural context?

    A. Reviewing the client's family photo album together

    B. Noticing the condition of furniture in the client's apartment

    C. Meeting the client's best friend

    D. Befriending the client's dog who comes to greet you as you enter her apartment

28. Among the following interventions suited for vocational exploration, select the *first* activity that an OT could use with a male client who has an IQ of 70 and has no prior work history.
    A. Ask the client to list anticipated problems he thinks may occur on the job
    B. Ask the client to complete a sample job application
    C. Ask the client to perform a simulated job task and observe work skills
    D. Ask the client to role play interview techniques

29. Choose the OT intervention that is *best* suited to foster self-management for a client who is coping with an incident of sexual assault.
    A. Identify emotional triggers and list new cognitive strategies to modify behaviors
    B. Identify a list of values that relate to one's physical, emotional, and sexual self
    C. Identify one's primary roles in life and evaluate effectiveness of their functions
    D. Identify effective verbal and nonverbal skills to be used with persons in authority

30. What OT intervention is *best* suited to increase self-acceptance with a female adolescent client who has bulimia?
    A. Attend a social dance with a friend of her choice
    B. Volunteer to work with children who have special needs
    C. Create a self-portrait using materials of the client's choice
    D. Run for president of her class

31. Select the *most* objective assessment strategy to use with an adolescent who is disruptive in a classroom and has poor time management, poor academic performance, and poor impulse control.
    A. An interview with the adolescent
    B. A structured observation of the adolescent in the classroom
    C. Completion of a self-inventory concerning occupational performance
    D. Attending a case conference at school (IEP) and consulting with the team

32. Select the *most* effective occupational intervention for a 10-year-old female in fifth grade. She has no identified friends, has poor social skills, and subsequently has low confidence in herself.
    A. Joining Girl Scouts
    B. Taking piano lessons
    C. Working as a volunteer in a daycare center
    D. Exercising to video tapes

33. The following are contraindications for giving an elderly person a rocker knife *except:*
    A. Limited range of motion in the upper extremity
    B. Tremors
    C. Cognitive impairments
    D. Lack of strong grip

34. Which documentation procedure is likely to be challenged in a malpractice lawsuit?
    A. Patient response to evaluation
    B. Signatures that are legible
    C. Progress notes charted at the end of the day
    D. Records not fraudulently altered

35. Which approach is *least* effective in managing negative behaviors in brain injury rehabilitation?
    A. Work with the patient one-to-one in a quiet room
    B. Provide correct information when the patient does not know the information
    C. Expect the patient to participate in his or her rehabilitation by allowing him or her to select simple, meaningful activities
    D. Use simple words and sentences, allow processing time, and repeat if necessary

36. An OT is presenting a workshop at the local OT conference. The OT wants to make copies of an article from the national association's journal to give to participants. What issue is *most* important?
    A. Copyright infringement—the OT must have permission from the journal to make copies
    B. Copyright fair use—the OT can make limited copies because it is a nonprofit conference
    C. Copyright permission—the OT can make unlimited copies because she is a member of the national association that publishes the journal
    D. Copyright registration—the OT can check to see if the article is registered

37. Which is *most* effective in preventing contractures?
    A. Positioning
    B. Therapeutic exercise
    C. Serial casting
    D. Splinting

38. What is the focus of treatment for children with Rett syndrome?
    A. Increase tone
    B. Decrease stereotypic hand movements
    C. Decrease spasticity and ataxia
    D. Decrease rocking behaviors

39. What type of clothing do people with disabilities generally prefer?
    A. Slip-on type with no closures
    B. Fabrics that hold their shape and do not stretch
    C. Velcro closures on any type clothing
    D. Clothing sold based on their disability

40. What type of splint can control swan neck deformities and meet emotional issues?
    A. Small serial casting splints in bright thermoplastics
    B. Resting hand splint with Velcro closures in the color chosen by the client
    C. Silver ring splints
    D. Dynamic extension alignment splint

41. Which handwriting tool would be *least* effective in a home program for elementary school-age children?
    A. Exercise putty
    B. Slant board
    C. Assorted manipulatives
    D. Hair gel in a plastic zipper bag

42. Superficial heat agents are contraindicated for which condition?
    A. Stiff joints
    B. Muscle spasms
    C. Chronic arthritis
    D. Deep vein thrombophlebitis

43. What treatment option for a person with hemiplegia shoulder subluxation is *least* effective in controlling edema?
    A. Slings or shoulder taping
    B. Lapboard
    C. Arm trough
    D. Bilateral rolling platform walker

44. When is an OT responsible for "duty to warn"?
    A. A patient is threatening bodily harm to another person
    B. An elderly person is being abused
    C. A child is being abused by an adult
    D. All of the above

45. What is the recommended slope for ramps to be added to an existing home to make it accessible to a person with a spinal cord injury?
    A. 6 inches of length for every 1 inch of height
    B. 12 inches of length for every 1 inch of height
    C. 18 inches of length for every 1 inch of height
    D. Whatever fits the property

46. All of the following supportive and compensatory strategies are effective in treating a person with low vision *except:*
    A. Eye patch
    B. Modify lighting
    C. Increase contrast
    D. Teach the use of visual markers

47. An effective fieldwork supervisor does all of the following *except:*
    A. Has a broad knowledge base
    B. Critiques constructively
    C. Has the supervisee figure it out on his or her own
    D. Takes time to explain in the present

48. An OT has recently been hired to replace an OT who moved out of state. Management has asked for a quality assurance report for the last 3 months. The former OT never collected the data needed, and the data cannot be collected retrospectively. What should the OT do *first*?
    A. Notify management that the data are not available and ask how the situation should be handled
    B. Notify management that the data are not available and present an alternative plan to retrospectively collect QA data
    C. Notify management that the data are not available and report the former OT to appropriate state or national organizations for possible ethical violations
    D. Collect new data related to the current QA question and report that data to management

49. Intervention goals can include all of the following *except:*
    A. Occurrence of pain-free performance
    B. Gradation to more complex performance
    C. Improved quality of performance
    D. Assessment performance results

50. All of the following *Standards of Practice* can be done by both OTs and OTAs *except:*
    A. Educate referral sources about scope of services
    B. Follow defined protocols when standardized assessments are used
    C. Maintain or seek current information relevant to the client's needs
    D. Document recommendations for discharge follow-up or reevaluation

Section Two Answers and Explanations

1. Answer: D

Deficits caused by a learning disability affect short-term memory, which may be used for spelling and reading. Memory may then heighten the ADHD symptoms. The other areas may be appropriate assessment for a student, but memory must be addressed first.

2. Answer: C

Gout is a condition of hyperuricemia, typically affecting the great toe but not limited to this joint. Acute swelling and painful, hot joints result. Gout is exacerbated by alcohol ingestion (especially beer), obesity, and low urine volume. Some medications also affect the condition, so the client should also inform the doctor of other medications he is taking.

3. Answer: A

Snacking and juice throughout the day will mean the child is not hungry at mealtime. Picky eaters, especially toddlers, have special issues. First, many toddlers are picky eaters and this passes with time. Toddlers are experimenting with the word "no" and often try this during meals. The child must trust the feeder, and other emotional needs must be met. The OT can model positive feeding behaviors if needed. Age-appropriate portions are often one-third to one-fourth an adult portion. Play during feeding can reduce stress and increase trust.

4. Answer: C

Using a mirror for the baby to lift her head is most appropriate for the prone position. The other activities encourage reach.

5. Answer: A

Needs assessment is part of program development. Environmental assessment is examining the population served. Organizational assessment evaluates its effectiveness with the population. Market analysis is the use of information from the environmental and organizational assessments.

6. Answer: A

The ball allows for increased sensory input so that the student can stay focused on the task at his desk. The other chairs are restrictive and would not change the problem. There is no indication that there is a motor issue.

7. Answer: A

All the tests are appropriate for driver's evaluation, but the OT should begin the evaluation with an interview to establish rapport, judge insight, discover the driver's perception of problems, and generally assess functioning levels.

8. Answer: D

Collaboration with other people for the common good is beneficial; however, lobbyists are trained professionals who have the ears of senators and congress people who make changes in laws. A primary function of AOTA (and where member dues are used) is to advocate for the profession at the national and state legislative levels.

9. Answer: D

The OT knows that she is medically stable before transfer to rehabilitation. Although an assessment of her functioning in the acute setting may be interesting, it likely will be of little assistance to her functioning after rehabilitation. Environmental changes require social support and may include financial issues depending on the resources of the client.

10. Answer: B

Personal questions are illegal. Only questions related to the job can be asked.

11. Answer: C

The KELS is a measure of performance areas. The other three assessments are appropriate for dementia but measure cognitive performance components.

12. Answer: D

The neck should be in neutral.

13. Answer: C

Walking the tongue depressor toward the back of the tongue will desensitize the gag reflex. When possible the patient should control the tongue depressor while the therapist observes. Icing is an exercise for muscle strength. Resistance to the jaw is for jaw control. Increasing straw length is effective for the sucking reflex.

14. Answer: B

If possible, have the patient apply pressure himself. If not, the OT should don a latex glove, put a gauze on the cut, and apply pressure. Return the patient to his unit and notify the nurse. Fill out the appropriate incident report forms.

15. Answer: D

Mobile arm supports are effective in proximal weakness. Although A, B, and C may be helpful, they are designed for distal weakness.

16. Answer: B

Hepatitis will affect the patient's ability to participate in the rehabilitation program. Diazepam (Valium) may cause seizures. Baclofen may cause hallucinations, and clonidine may cause a decrease in blood pressure.

17. Answer: D

Part of energy conservation is planning ahead to pace oneself and save energy.

18. Answer: B

Using informal methods until the teenager is more comfortable with the therapist is best. Other responses are likely to further agitate the teen.

19. Answer: C

The patient with a T-4 spinal cord injury can use a wheelchair with removable sides to transfer in and out of the chair. If a patient is confused or agitated, removable sides on a wheelchair would be dangerous.

20. Answer: C

A demonstration may help the patient understand what it is that you want him to do. A, B, and D will only further agitate the patient.

21. Answer: A

Patients dealing with or recovering from cancer have diverse needs, often including most of the areas of *The Practice Framework*. Prognosis, treatments, and medications are the expertise of the physician. Encourage the patient to ask her doctor. If she is unable to do this independently, assist her in developing the needed skills or refer her to someone who can advocate for her.

22. Answer: B

This is a monitoring plan. A, C, and D are all indicators of quality programs.

23. Answer: B

Diversion activities assist persons to focus their attention away from the anxiety and onto a substitute source. This diverting of attention has been shown to decrease anxiety and regulate autonomic responses. Mental health interventions provide strategies for managing and restoring function, rather than providing a cure for symptoms.

24. Answer: B

The definition of time management is the planning and involvement in self-care, work, leisure, and rest for personal satisfaction. Self-concept includes one's personal values about physical, emotional, and sexual aspects. Self-expression includes the use of various forms of communication to reveal thoughts, feelings, and needs. Self-control is the ability to adapt one's behavior to match the needs and expectations of the environment.

25. Answer: B

Restoring a deficit in a performance component is an intervention used by occupational therapists. Answers A, C, and D are not based on occupational performance but are more related to the medical model of treatment.

26. Answer: C

Competence refers to a person's ability to demonstrate skills based on the demands of his or her environment. Meal preparation, an aspect of work/productive activities can *best* be assessed in the client's environmental context. Answers A and B will offer observation about task skill performance, and they do not take place in the client's preferred environment. Answer D is a performance area in activities of daily living, not work/productive activity.

27. Answer: A

Culture refers to customs, beliefs, activity patterns, and norms that are accepted by a particular group of persons sharing a common bond. Observing pictures and encouraging a client to tell the occupational therapist stories of the significant events, traditions, and rituals is a form of narrative reasoning that would reveal cultural standards. Answers B and D are aspects of the physical environmental context. Answer C is an example of a social context.

28. Answer: C

Vocational exploration involves determining a client's aptitudes, interests, and skills in order to select an appropriate vocational pursuit. Observing and assessing a client's work skills can be accomplished by both standardized and unstandardized testing procedures. The OT already knows some information about the client's cognitive ability by his IQ score, which puts him in the mild cognitive deficit range of functioning. Answer A is a reflective activity that requires higher level cognitive reasoning and may not match this client's reasoning capacity, especially since he has never worked before. Answers B and D are good interventions that could be given to this client following an assessment of his work abilities and a determination of the actual jobs at which this client may succeed.

29. Answer: A

Self-management includes having effective coping skills, time management, and self-control. Answer A includes the assessment of one's ability to cope and learn how to modify one's behavior to increase self-control. Answer B is related to the psychological component of self-concept. Answer C is related to the social component of role performance. Answer D is related to the social component of interpersonal skills.

30. Answer: C

Self-acceptance is the ability to be pleased with oneself in the absence of external feedback from others. Answer C is the only activity that is self-directed and focused. All of the other activities include interaction and feedback from the environment.

31. Answer: B

A structured observation by the OT in the natural environment will provide the most objective data regarding the identified problems. Answers A and C will provide the adolescent's subjective experience. Answer D will provide information that has been gathered by other disciplines and members of the team. All four answers are appropriate as part of the assessment process because each serves to give information from a unique perspective. An effective OT will compare all the data and use clinical reasoning skills to ascertain what is problematic for this student.

32. Answer: A

A major developmental task of this age group is the need to belong and be accepted by peers. Social functioning is a common deficit area for children with psychosocial dysfunction. Socialization at this age is learned predominantly by peer interaction rather than adult intervention. A structured group and/or organization, such as Girl Scouts, will allow the opportunity for this client to learn and experiment with social behaviors among a group of peers. Answers B and D are both solitary types of activities and do not allow for peer association. Answer C is not a realistic and developmentally suited role for this client's developmental stage.

33. Answer: A

Limited ROM is an indicator for a rocker knife. All the other answers are safety concerns for a rocker knife.

34. Answer: C

Documentation principles include objective patient response to evaluation and treatment, follow-up instructions to family and friends, notations that are timely and legible, and records that are never tampered with. An attorney will question how a staff member could remember each patient's response after treating eight to 10 different patients.

35. Answer: C

People with head injuries may not be able to make choices and may seem resistive to rehabilitation. A quiet, supportive, reassuring environment that can be processed by the person is most effective. As healing progresses, participation in the rehabilitation process will improve.

36. Answer: A

The OT must request copyright permission to make copies from a journal or she is breaking copyright laws. Fair use is generally understood to be one copy for personal use. Registration is a moot point because any copies need the publisher's or author's permission. It should be noted that permission to copy is often very easy to get, especially for educational purposes. When the copies are to be sold for profit, the copyright holder usually requires a small fee.

37. Answer: A

All the answers are effective treatments for contractures, including the addition of physical agent modalities. Once reduced, contractures can be avoided with correct positioning to encourage normalized tone.

38. Answer: B

Rett syndrome affects females beginning at age 8 months. Stereotypic hand movements include hand wringing, hand to head, and hand to mouth behaviors, leaving the child unable to play. Initially, hypotonia is present but later spasticity develops. The loss of purposeful hand movements limits the child's attention to play and leads to developmental issues. The hand movements are the focus of treatment.

39. Answer: A

A research study found that people with disabilities preferred clothes without closures and that slipped on. Velcro-type fasteners were frustrating because they "looked disabled," felt rough, caught on clothes, and filled with lint. Participants reported they wanted soft clothes with stretch that made them feel warm. In general, they bought clothes for the same reason as nondisabled people, "to look good."

40. Answer: C

Silver ring splints are attractive jewelry that hold joints in extension. They can be worn on every finger. The other splints may be appropriate, but they look like medical devices.

41. Answer: B

All the tools are effective with the addition of squeeze toys and vibrating pens. A slant board might be used with some families, but because of the size, it might not be practical for storage.

42. Answer: D

Superficial heat may be helpful for stiff joints, chronic arthritis, muscle spasms, and contractures but is contraindicated for DVT, tumors, impaired sensation, infections, and rheumatoid arthritis.

43. Answer: A

Taping or slings can control for subluxation but do not assist in edema control because the hand remains in a lower position.

44. Answer: D

Although there are not any "all of the above" questions on the NBCOT exam, this answer is meant to educate the reader about the legal responsibility of duty to warn. Duty to warn means a practitioner must notify legal parties when a person or the public is at risk, even when it means breaking confidentiality. Each state and some local counties have their own rules, but abuse or bodily harm must be reported in all states.

45. Answer: B

Twelve inches in length for every inch in height; however, outside ramps are longer (up to 20 inches) for every inch up.

46. Answer: A

Eye patching is a direct remediation for strabismic binocular vision disorders. Low vision does not respond to direct remediation. The other answers are effective compensatory interventions.

47. Answer: C

A good supervisor generates alternatives when the supervisee is struggling. This inspires confidence and trust in the relationship.

48. Answer: B

Notify management of the problem and possible plan. Next, the OT should review state licensure laws and national organization code of ethics and report any possible violations.

49. Answer: D

Assessment results are used to develop goals and are not reported in the goal section of documentation. Assessment results might be considered a baseline data set that could be integrated into goals. All the other answers are appropriate for intervention goals. Goals should be linked to *The Practice Framework*. Further examples can be found in Moyers' 1999 *Guide to Occupational Therapy Practice*.

50. Answer: D

The OT is responsible for this area. Both OTAs and OTs can complete the tasks in the other three answers. The *Official Documents* (AOTA, 2004) and the *Guide to Occupational Therapy Practice* (Moyers, 1999) can provide further information.

Section Three Domain-Style Questions

1. Assessment of client performance can be contaminated by the following:
   A. Infectious material at the test site
   B. The OT cueing the client
   C. Hazards specifically added to the testing for evaluation
   D. The OT following the standard administration

2. When assessing home safety, staging hazards in the home evaluation can provide effective feedback to the team, family, and client. The OT must *first* use:
   A. Real hazards to simulate problems in the home
   B. Photos of hazards to have the client identify
   C. Judgment in deciding which hazards should be set up
   D. Cueing to the client

3. A person at the highest level of cognitive functioning following recovery from a head injury may still need some assistance to be modified independent in the following situation:
   A. Handling multiple tasks with breaks
   B. Completing familiar household tasks
   C. Keeping memory devices
   D. When sick, fatigued, or under stress

4. The *best* way to develop professional competencies throughout an OT's career is:
   A. Attend conferences
   B. Return to school for more education
   C. Network with peers
   D. Develop a professional development plan

5. The *first* issue to be addressed in a community-based early intervention program for children with disabilities is:
   A. Play and play exploration
   B. Collaboration with family members
   C. Functional toileting
   D. Feeding

6. While doing a kitchen activity in a home evaluation, the client spills a glass of juice off the counter and begins to clean it up. What should the OT do *next*?
   A. Stand by to grab the gait belt
   B. Tell the client to stop, the OT will clean up the spill
   C. Have the client safely sit while the OT cleans to the spill
   D. Move to a safer section of the kitchen until the spill can be cleaned

7. Concerned over a unique clinical situation, the OT has completed an evidence-based practice research of the literature. The OT has reviewed the material and established a treatment plan. What is the *next* step in the process?
   A. Discuss the research with the client in language free of professional jargon
   B. Notify the client of the treatment plan
   C. Gather the necessary supplies need for the treatment approach
   D. Notify the treatment team of the new approach

8. While recovering from an illness or accident, the client may also be recovering from:
   A. Loss of occupations resulting from the illness or accident
   B. Loss of income related to the illness or accident
   C. Medication side effects
   D. All of the above

9. All of the following are primary areas of occupation for children in an early intervention setting *except*:
   A. Functional mobility
   B. Social participation
   C. Handwriting
   D. Toileting

10. An entry-level OT is concerned about a client's driving skill and is questioning if a referral should be made to a driving specialist. The OT should *first* evaluate:
    A. Mobility alternatives such as public transportation
    B. Range of motion, vision, cognitive functioning
    C. The client's behind-the-wheel skills
    D. How open the client is to counseling

11. The *most* effective treatment for cumulative trauma disorders is:
    A. Rest from the activity that caused the problem
    B. Splints to immobilize
    C. Reduce edema
    D. Client education and activity modification

12. The Health Insurance Portability and Accountability Act of 1996 (HIPAA, but sometimes called HIPPA) covers the administration and fraud of insurance. This law requires OTs have written permission from the patient before disclosing information of all of the following *except*:
    A. Providing treatment
    B. Obtaining payment
    C. Carrying out health care operations
    D. Talking with the potential patients

13. A mother of a child the OT has been treating in a preschool program has become frustrated by her child's "escapes from the car seat" while she is driving. What is the *best* recommendation?
    A. Behavioral techniques applied each time the child gets out of the car restraint
    B. A car seat with better positioning and support
    C. A vest that fastens in the back and tethers to the seat belt
    D. A companion to sit with the child in the back seat

14. A client with a vestibular disorder is referred to the OT clinic for treatment. When the OT greets her she immediately states, "The doctor says you are going to make me dizzy as part of my treatment!" What would be the *best* approach?
    A. Reassure the client that she may be dizzy but will be safe
    B. Explain that you will be repositioning any dislodged otoliths to stop the dizziness
    C. State that many clients feel uneasy about moving and that this fear will be addressed before any treatment starts
    D. Explain that activities will be graded before advancing to the next level

15. Medications that might affect balance in clients include all of the following *except*:
    - A. Anti-psychotic
    - B. Anti-depressive
    - C. Hypertension
    - D. High cholesterol

16. A 4-year-old with developmental issues is working on developing finger control as a foundation to begin writing. The child enjoys active play independently but still has some behavioral issues that do not allow unsupervised play. All of the following fine motor activities would be good choices *except*:
    - A. Putting coins in and out of a piggy bank
    - B. Play dough art
    - C. Paper airplanes
    - D. Large refrigerator magnets

17. Brushing with a surgical brush is a treatment technique for overresponsiveness to sensory stimuli. This technique administers:
    - A. Direct deep-touch pressure
    - B. Light superficial-touch pressure
    - C. Improved circulation to the skin
    - D. Alternating alerting and calming responses

18. Elder abuse in an institution might be manifested by all of the following *except*:
    - A. Lack of occupational therapy services
    - B. Persons left unattended on the toilet
    - C. Shortage of care staff on nights or weekends
    - D. Bedsores on buttock, heels, or elbows

19. Appropriate environmental adaptations for visual impairments include all of the following *except*:
    - A. Remove low coffee tables or magazine racks
    - B. Place colored tape on a cane to make it easy to find
    - C. Mark stair treads with high contrast edges
    - D. Improve lighting in common pathways

20. Work tolerance screenings can be completed after an applicant has been given a conditional employment offer. During this screening, the occupational therapy practitioner can offer:
    - A. A final employment offer
    - B. Advice to the applicant about his or her job performance
    - C. Reasonable accommodation options to complete the job
    - D. A prediction of future effectiveness on the job

21. A functional reach screening shows the client is unable to move body parts independent of each other. The *next* area to assess is:
    - A. Endurance
    - B. Reflex testing
    - C. Strength
    - D. Postural control

22. A referral from a home care provider states concern for the client's cognitive and perceptual skills. An assessment in this area includes all of the following *except*:
    A. Insight and awareness
    B. Orientation and attention
    C. Visual motor
    D. Neuromuscular endurance

23. A client having difficulty organizing and problem solving would benefit from further assessment of:
    A. Executive functioning
    B. Orientation
    C. Insight and judgment
    D. Affect and mood

24. A client would need to have what forward reach to access items on a standard kitchen counter?
    A. 12 inches
    B. 18 inches
    C. 21 inches
    D. 32 inches

25. What environmental adaptation would allow a wheelchair user to garden effectively?
    A. Watering wand to extend the hose
    B. Raised garden bed
    C. Extended reach garden tools
    D. Built-up handle garden tools

26. During a home evaluation following sub-acute rehabilitation services for a CVA, the OT notices the client is unable to reach the toilet paper without balance issues. What is the *best* recommendation?
    A. Use a reacher already provided to the client
    B. Install grab bars for positioning on the toilet
    C. Substitute a free-standing toilet tissue holder that can be moved
    D. Install a commode near the bed

27. A client is experiencing sensory problems following a peripheral nerve injury that is interfering with his ability to return to work as an assembly line worker. He is receiving sensory reeducation as part of his therapy. What issue is addressed *last*?
    A. Hypersensitivity
    B. Scar tissue formation
    C. Strengthening
    D. Stereognosis

28. Which techniques could inhibit negative motor responses in a client with excess tone and limited participation in ADLs?
    A. Joint compression
    B. Icing
    C. Quick stretch
    D. Light moving touch

29. When positioning a client in bed lying on back, involved side, or uninvolved side using NDT principles to manage tone, which is true?

    A. Proximal musculature is positioned after the distal

    B. A head pillow is not used

    C. The head is supported with a pillow at midline

    D. Clients can maintain these positions for extended times because of pillow use

30. When training a client with unilateral neglect using visual scanning, which factor is *most* important?

    A. Visual preciseness

    B. Speed of eye movements

    C. Awareness of affected side

    D. Visual acuity

31. Which is true when adjusting a car seat for a child with a disability?

    A. Harness straps should have zero slack

    B. Head straps decrease the likelihood of injury

    C. Attached toys to the seat helps the child entertain himself or herself

    D. Padding can be added for additional support

32. All of the following are important concepts in pain management *except*:

    A. Clients learning to attend to the pain

    B. Relaxation techniques

    C. Increased physical activity

    D. Social support

33. Recline and tilt wheelchairs provide for all of the following *except*:

    A. Relief of pressure

    B. Posture management

    C. Added comfort

    D. Active mobility for low-level injuries

34. Under Medicare Part B rules group therapy rates must be charged if:

    A. The patient is seen individually but the family is present

    B. Two clients are treated individually but at the same therapist's time

    C. The therapist is giving direct therapy services

    D. Any consultation services are provided

35. A home care client with diabetes begins to complain that he is not feeling well with sweating, shakiness, and fast pulse. The OT stops treatment and:

    A. Calls 911 as these are symptoms of a heart attack

    B. Makes arrangements for the next appointment when the client feels better

    C. Has the client test his blood sugar level and if under 110, have a snack

    D. Has the client test his blood sugar level and if under 70, have a snack

36. A client in treatment for breast cancer is experiencing the common side effects of chemotherapy including fatigue, loss of appetite, mouth sores, and common infections. She asks the OT to include complementary therapies in her approach to treatment. The OT agrees and does all of the following *except*:
    A. Focus on the complementary treatments that support long-term goals in OT
    B. Documents intervention so client's progress can be measured
    C. Seeks additional information from magazines and health food experts
    D. Adds breathing, relaxation, guided imagery, aromatherapy, and massage to treatment

37. Occupations of a newborn infant or premature baby in a neonatal intensive care unit include all of the following *except*:
    A. Sleeping
    B. Social interaction
    C. Procuring
    D. Feeding

38. What type of splint is preferred after trauma or surgery that involves an open wound?
    A. Commercial
    B. Modified prefabricated
    C. Precut
    D. Custom

39. Occupational therapy intervention for carpal tunnel syndrome includes all of the following *except*:
    A. Sensory testing
    B. Electrodiagnostics
    C. Functional loss evaluation
    D. Neuromuscular imbalance assessment

40. Sara Anne is an elderly woman living in a church community that values conservative family values. Although she has elderly friends in the area she does not have any family except for sisters 150 miles away. The social worker is concerned that Sara Anne is at risk of a serious fall as she has had several "trips." The OT evaluation shows a woman who rarely leaves her apartment, is sometimes confused or dizzy, and reports being fatigued. What would be the OT's *next* approach?
    A. Refer her to her family medical doctor
    B. Address her fear of falling with counseling
    C. Educate her about home hazards
    D. Evaluate visual problems

41. Diabetic retinopathy can cause loss of vision from retinal bleeding. Functional activities must consider all of the following *except*:
    A. Avoid heavy lifting
    B. Avoid bending head below heart level
    C. Avoid exercise and stretching
    D. Avoid holding breath or straining

42. Henry is an outpatient client with numerous medical conditions including post CVA, heart disease, long-term diabetes, low vision, and arthritis. He is a war veteran who took up smoking in the military service and has not stopped. He wears heavy eyeglasses and is unsure in his gait. He typically has a list of complaints when he arrives for his appointment. Counseling skills are appropriate intervention for all of the following complaints *except*:

    A. Stiffness in the morning when he wakes up
    B. Blurry vision and "things" floating in his vision
    C. Left hand weakness since his CVA
    D. Lack of friends since "they are all gone"

43. A client is referred to OT services for a functional assessment following a diagnosis of fibromyalgia syndrome. She reports both frustration and relief as it took 4 years for a "proper diagnosis." She has adjusted her life as she coped with "that unknown thing" but would like to sleep better so she has more energy during the day with her 4-year-old. The OT helps the client establish sleep routines and habits by recommending all of the following *except*:

    A. Set aside some play time with the 4-year-old each evening
    B. Limit activities in bed to sleeping and sex
    C. Add aerobic exercise each day
    D. Add strength training to her exercise routine

Use the following information to answer questions 44 and 45: A recent immigrant family has been referred to an outpatient clinic to address their daughter's preschool skills as she has spastic cerebral palsy. The parents were political refugees and are very happy to be in a new country, eager to help their children, but guarded about outside people. There are some language barriers and a translator is not always available. The mother states she wants her children to be successful in school and grow up "strong and independent."

44. Range of motion is limited in the child's UE as the political nature of her parents forbid treatment in her former country. With hand use as an important family goal, the OT recommends:

    A. Passive range of motion
    B. Active range of motion
    C. Active assistive range of motion
    D. Serial inhibitory casting

45. The OT is concerned that the casting might be worrisome to the family because its appearance of restraints, something the family has reported from their former country. All of the following is appropriate to educating the family about the option of casting *except*:

    A. Demonstrate on the child
    B. Write a description of the process and have a translator explain it to the family
    C. Have the family meet another family who is using this treatment method
    D. Use counseling techniques after explaining the process to the family

46. A child with spina bifida at the sacral level is being screened as part of the normal preregistration process of entering kindergarten. The child had been seen by OTs and PTs in preschool programs but is currently not receiving services. The OT expects to see what level of sensorimotor impairments?

    A. Variable weakness/loss from the waist down
    B. Paralysis of lower legs but some movement of hip and legs
    C. Weak foot flexion and some hip problems but all other leg movements
    D. Mild weakness in lower leg

47. Social skills training is often used with people with serious and persistent mental health disorders. The OT should use all of the following strategies *except*:
    A. Avoid feedback, allowing the client to self-evaluate performance
    B. Provide opportunities to practice skills in real life situations
    C. Use motivators and rewards that match the skills being taught
    D. Individualize education to the cognitive level of the client

48. Elastic garments and inserts are effective at scar control following burns, however, splints may be more effective in certain body areas including:
    A. Neck, face, and mouth
    B. Chest and back
    C. Lower abdomen
    D. Knees and elbows

49. As the OT providing services to a community living program that services the elderly with mental retardation, you have been asked to inservice the staff about hip precautions in preparation for the return of a resident who fell and broke his hip while gardening. Hip precautions include all of the following *except*:
    A. Crossing legs at ankles
    B. Crossing the legs at knees
    C. Hip flexion beyond 90 degrees
    D. Knee full extension

50. The OT in the above situation is concerned that the resident will want to sleep on the unaffected hip because he likes facing the door in his bedroom and also watching his television. The OT is concerned because:
    A. The affected hip will not have support in the bed
    B. The affected hip will be the lead extremity when raising out of the bed
    C. This encourages internal rotation of the affected hip
    D. This leaves the incision exposed

Section Three Answers and Explanations

1. Answer: B

A common problem in assessment is the OT providing cues to the client. The occupational therapist must remember that assessment is not treatment and should follow the standard administration directions without providing assistance.

2. Answer: C

Hazards can be excellent ways to assess a client's performance in his or her home, however, the OT's judgment is most important.

3. Answer: D

A person at RLA level X (10) is able to complete A, B, and C without assistance but may become frustrated and irritable when tired or ill.

4. Answer: D

There are many ways to develop professional competencies including A, B, and C. A professional development plan is an individualized map to achieving these skills. In addition, this plan assists the OT in documenting skills to outside reviewers.

5. Answer: B

Collaboration with family will establish the occupations of the child and his or her current developmental level. The other answers may be appropriate following collaboration.

6. Answer: A

While safety is always first and the OT must make a clinical judgment, this is a home evaluation and the client is likely to face this same situation without the OT being available. Since cleaning a spill on the floor requires bending, the gait belt on the client before the evaluation begins will help the client be safe in cleaning the spill.

7. Answer: A

The evidence-based practice approach includes consulting with the client about what was found in the literature and how it might apply to the client. After agreement from all involved, the OT would move forward to the treatment stage.

8. Answer: D

Although there are no "all of the above" answers on the NBCOT exam, this question is designed to educate the reader to the multi-faceted nature of recovery.

9. Answer: C

Handwriting may be addressed as pre-handwriting skills, however, it is typically addressed in the school system once the child has begun formal school. ADLs, play, and social participation are occupations of children from birth to age 3.

10. Answer: B

The other areas are also of concern to the OT, however, a basic evaluation of performance would be helpful in establishing the next step in driving.

11. Answer: D

All the answers are appropriate treatment for cumulative trauma disorders as well as heat or ice, however, only D addresses the issue of reoccurring trauma.

12. Answer: D

HIPAA is a complicated law designed to protect patient records. The administration of the facility has likely addressed this issue to ensure timely payments from funding sources once treatment begins. An OT can talk to potential clients about services available but would still be required to hold any information disclosed confidentially under state laws and the AOTA code of ethics.

13. Answer: C

Although behavioral techniques might work, the mother may not be able to apply the techniques while driving. A car seat addressing positioning and support is best for the child with limited trunk control. A companion might be effective but may not be available. As safety is always the most important issue, the vest that closes in the back would be the safe option.

14. Answer: C

Clients with dizziness will be very guarded about moving and forming relationships with therapists they think might make them dizzy. Although all the answers might be true, addressing the fear is the first issue. Answers B and D have professional jargon the person might not understand.

15. Answer: D

A, B, and C might have balance issues or falls as side effects of the medication. Statins, commonly used for cholesterol, are known to cause problems with balance.

16. Answer: A

Although this is a fine motor activity, small coins or paper clips could be placed in the mouth and cause a safety issue. The other items might also be placed in the mouth but are bigger than coins.

17. Answer: A

This technique, know as the Wilbarger Protocol, uses deep pressure to calm overresponsiveness.

18. Answer: A

Although a facility would benefit by having OT services, this is not an automatic warning sign of possible abuse as many institutions service clients who might not benefit from direct services. All the other issues as well as poor hygiene, inadequate dental hygiene, unexplained weight loss, or persons in soiled beds are signs of neglect.

19. Answer: B

Although an excellent treatment approach, marking a cane is adapting an assistive device. Environmental modifications include all of the other answers plus any task that alters the living situation.

20. Answer: C

The screener can offer accommodations to assess how the applicant performs the tasks of the job. A, B, and D should not be offered. A full ergonomic assessment might provide additional information and can be suggested in the screening process.

21. Answer: D

Postural control seems to be the issue related to the coordination of reach. The other areas should be assessed as well, but an understanding of postural adaptation is the first issue to address.

22. Answer: D

Cognition and perception are interrelated processes required to see and use information in our daily lives. Endurance is a physical process that might affect cognitive functioning when low but is not part of the cognitive-perceptual assessment of a client. In addition to A, B, and C, visual processing, unilateral neglect, memory, and motor planning are assessed.

23. Answer: A

Organization and problem solving are upper level cognitive functioning skills. The ability to self-monitor is important to independence and should be further evaluated. The other areas mentioned might be appropriate to assess after executive functioning issues are addressed.

24. Answer: C

Standard kitchen counters are 21 inches deep, typically available to anyone who has full elbow extension and movement of the shoulder.

25. Answer: B

The other tools might be helpful, but the gardener wants to be able to touch the plants from a sitting position.

26. Answer: C

The reacher might be helpful in the house but will not work with tissue. Grab bars might be a good idea for balance but the issue is likely reach. An inexpensive standing tissue holder will address this and not look like adaptive equipment in the bath.

27. Answer: D̶ C

Strengthening might not be an issue. Before stereognosis can be addressed, especially for a worker who works on an assembly line, hypersensitivity and scar tissue must be addressed.

28. Answer: A

Slow rocking or stroking, deep tendon pressure, and joint compression inhibit while the others facilitate motor response.

29. Answer: C

All others are not true and can cause additional problems. Proximal motor control is addressed first to assist distal. The client's position must be moved a minimum of every 2 hours to avoid skin problems.

30. Answer: C

Lack of eye movements to the neglected side results in inattention.

31. Answer: A

Padding should never be added behind or under the child as this changes the straps' effectiveness. Head straps and attached toys increase the risk of injuries in an accident.

32. Answer: A

Cognitive restructuring and distraction are important aspects of pain management where a client learns to pull his or her attention away from the pain. Increased physical activity, relaxation, social support, stress management, and biofeedback are also helpful in the management of the pain.

33. Answer: D

Active users should have low back chairs for best mobility.

34. Answer: B

Group rates are charged when the OT is seeing two individual patients at the same time.

35. Answer: D

If blood sugar levels are under 70, this likely explains the symptoms which should be addressed with 15 g carbohydrates intake. This includes 4 oz fruit juice, sugared soda, or 8 oz lowfat milk. The client should test his blood sugar again 15 minutes later and if normal, return to therapy. Heart attack is always a possible issue with people with diabetes as they have high risk factors. If you are unsure, consult the doctor in charge of his care.

36. Answer: C

Information from magazines, experts, and health marketing tools are likely not evidence-based practice. The first rule of complementary therapists is first do no harm. The OT should use scientifically reviewed journal articles to research complementary therapies that are effective.

37. Answer: A

Sleeping is a passive activity and not considered an occupation, however, getting ready to sleep is an occupation. Social interaction with family and staff, making needs known (procuring), and feeding are occupations of an infant.

38. Answer: D

A custom splint allows for adjustments to open wounds. Some commercially available products may allow some modifications, however, this varies.

39. Answer: B

Electrodiagnostics is a medical test commonly done by the medical doctor for carpal tunnel syndrome. The other assessments are done by the OT and treatment may include exercises, inflammation management, and splinting with the goal of pain reduction.

40. Answer: A

Dizziness, confusion, and sleepiness might be due to medical conditions such as urinary tract infections, postural hypotension, dehydration, or medicine side effects. All the other answers are also appropriate after all medical issues have been ruled out.

41. Answer: C

Exercise and stretching are healthy as long as within medical limitations. Consult the client's eye doctor or general physician for limits on lifting weight, blood pressure, or bending.

42: Answer: B

Immediately contact the client's eye doctor about a sudden onset of "floaters." As this client has diabetes, he may be experiencing a decline in his vision.

43. Answer: A

Play in the evening will likely get the child and mom in an alert stage that will make sleep for both difficult. Quiet routines and habits in the evening will assist in preparing for sleep. Exercise and strengthening are helpful in sleep if done earlier in the day. The bed should be used only for sleep or sex. Reading, eating, or playing should not be done in bed if the goal is sleep improvement.

44. Answer: D

Serial inhibitory casting has been shown to increase hand function in children with cerebral palsy. Since language may be a problem, the range of motion options might be ineffective or contraindicated.

45. Answer: A

No casting should be done until the family and child understands the purpose and have discussed the issue of restraints especially since restraints are sometimes used as torture by some governments.

46. Answer: D

Answer A is thoracic, L-1, or L-2. Answer B is L-3. Answer C is L-4 or L-5.

47. Answer: A

Persons with serious mental health disorders are likely to have weaknesses in insight and judgment making internal feedback inaccurate. The OT should provide concrete feedback with specific examples of both positive and negative behaviors.

48. Answer: A

Early neck splinting prevents later issues of range of motion and the loss of the chin shelf. Face and mouth burns can cause problems with the lips and eating.

49. Answer: D

Knee extension is fine and used when the person must bend to pick something up. The effective hip is extended back, the knee is extended, and the unaffected hip is bent.

50. Answer: C

Internal rotation is not allowed in hip precautions. Placing the bed and television so the client does not roll on to his uninvolved side is important.

SECTION IV

Life After the Exam

Chapter Seven

Life After the Exam

Karen Sladyk, PhD, OTR/L, FAOTA, and Julie Seethaler, OTR/L

WAITING FOR THE RESULTS

Many occupational therapy students have said to us that waiting for the exam results is almost as hard as studying for the exam itself. Generally, you can expect the results by mail in approximately 3 weeks. Do not listen to rumors of how the results will look when you get them. We have heard that if the envelope has your name with OT next to it, you passed. We have also heard that if the envelope is thick, you passed. These rumors are not true. The only way to know if you passed the exam is to open the envelope.

WHAT IF YOU DID NOT PASS?

The percentage of people who do not pass the exam to become occupational therapists is about 15% to 20%. The reality is that some students will not pass, and one may be you. There are many reasons why students do not pass the exam. When they took the exam, some had major stressors in their life, such as a family illness or recent death. There are students who did well in school but may not be good test takers. Some students did not prepare for the exam by reviewing their weaker areas but simply reviewed their comfortable areas. Finally, there are those students who did not pass the exam and there is no clear-cut reason. Whatever the reason, it is our experience that you should not spend a lot of time ruminating over the fact that you did not pass. Of course, we realize that this is easy for us to say, and the bottom line is that not passing the exam hurts a lot.

What to Do First

If you have accepted a job offer or have already begun working, you will have to notify your employer. If possible, speak to the director of occupational therapy. The director will understand your problem better than the personnel department. Depending on the licensure laws in your state, you may be able to keep your job working as an occupational therapy aide or rehabilitation associate while studying for the next exam. Keep in mind that you do not want to practice occupational therapy until you have passed the exam due to liability concerns.

Other than the licensing board in your state, who will receive your scores from the NBCOT, no one else has access to your exam. We recommend that you share information about not passing with those who can be supportive as you study for the next exam. It is important to know that your school does not know who did not pass the exam unless you tell them.

After you have notified your employer, you should check with the appropriate people for further information about working and studying. These people may include:

- The testing center for hand correcting the exam you took
- The program director at your school
- The state licensing board for occupational therapists for further questions
- Your friends from school
- Other OTs who can help you study weak areas
- Other professors you found helpful or supportive in school

Lastly, we would like to discuss the emotional aspects of not passing the exam. It is our experience that this is a strong factor on how students cope with studying for the next exam. Not passing the exam the first time around will seem like a major loss in your life. It is expected that you deal with this loss in the same way that people usually deal with stressors. You can expect feelings of shock, anger, depression, and bargaining at first. Acceptance and coping will come later. Again, it is our experience that everyone does cope and is able to sit for the next exam. Generally, 2 months is enough time to develop coping skills. If coping is more difficult for you, seek professional help to deal with stress. We believe that counseling or therapy is one of the best treats you can give yourself. Do not be afraid or feel guilty for seeking professional help. Your college counseling center can provide you with a list of local supports. There is a 90-day waiting period between test and retest.

How to Get Going Again

Keep in mind that you are not the only one who has not passed the exam this time. You are not the first one, nor will you be the last one. It is important to keep things in perspective to increase your ability to cope. The following is a letter from an OT who did not pass the exam the first time.

To all students and future occupational therapists:

At this point in my life, I think it is important for me to share my personal story with you. My teachers in college would have described me as an above average student, but I worked hard to get there. During my last affiliation, with much resistance and procrastination, I began to study for the OT boards. When the day arrived to take the exam, I was quite anxious. When I walked out, it was hard to know how I did, but I was confident I had passed. Ironically, I consoled a friend and classmate who was confident she had failed.

After waiting 4 long weeks, I received the results. I had failed. I kept staring at the words "you did not meet the requirements..." Not only that but there was an address to reapply. I was supposed to be celebrating. They told us in school that "everyone passes" (or at least that was my perception). Despite many sad days and feeling unmotivated to try again, I got the books out and studied. When I looked back, I realized that I had studied the information I knew and was comfortable with instead of focusing on my weak areas of practice.

This time I did my preparation differently. I studied in a group. I reviewed with peers. I used a review book that provided me with structure. Lastly, I studied for many hours on my own. I focused only on my areas of weakness.

One thing that is important to mention is that I always had a tremendous amount of support from my family and friends. With all the support, studying, and courage to try again, I finally passed the exam the following year.

Although statistics show a low percentage rate for failing the exam, it does happen. It happened to me. My best advice is don't give up. Do your best and use supportive people to help you through the challenge. Although initially it was devastating, in the end it was a tremendous personal growth experience for me. I am currently practicing occupational therapy in an area that I enjoy, and I'm proud to be an OT.

My goal with this letter is to let everyone know that if you fail, you are not a failure. Do not give up even though you will have a strong desire to do so.

Best wishes to everyone,

J.T.

MAKING A NEW PLAN

Once you are ready to start studying again, it is important to develop a personalized plan of action. Chapter Two of this book took you through the planning process. As an OT who did not pass the exam the first time, you may need some additional plans in place. Look carefully at what caused difficulty the first time; however, understand that you may never know for sure what went wrong on the first exam. Globally review all your class notes and focus on weak areas of practice.

Understand that periods of anxiety and sadness may creep back on you as you prepare to take the exam again. If you are a person who experiences test anxiety, taking the exam a second time will likely cause much stress. Consider a relaxation exercise or visualize yourself calmly taking the exam and passing. Begin and end each study period with a visualization of you taking the exam and all the information you have studied flowing from your brain, down your arm, and onto the keyboard. Feel yourself calm, relaxed, and happy.

IF YOU DO NOT PASS AGAIN

Should you not pass the exam for a second time, you need to know what options are available to you. We know some great practicing occupational therapists who have experienced this challenge. Again, do not give up. If in your heart you know that occupational therapy is for you, do a thorough self-assessment of what went wrong, seek the help you need, and prepare to take the exam again.

SUMMARY

Finding out that you did not pass the OT exam will bring many emotional and cognitive challenges to you. Developing coping skills and preparing for the exam often will lead to passing the exam the next time. A thorough self-assessment of what went wrong the first time will help you develop an action plan. Notifying your employer if you are working and developing a support network of people who can help you study may be an effective way of coping with the challenges. Learning and using relaxation exercises may also be helpful. Whatever your options, do not give up—develop your resources and use your supports.

Appendices

Appendix A

Annotated Bibliography and Resources Used to Develop Study Questions

Allen, C. K., Earhart, C. A., & Blue, T. (1992). *Occupational therapy treatment goals for the physically and cognitively disabled.* Bethesda, MD: American Occupational Therapy Association.
> Provides information on cognitive function, evaluation, and instruments. Performance analysis is reviewed in detail and suggestions for treatment are provided.

American Occupational Therapy Association. (2004). *Official documents of AOTA.* Bethesda, MD: Author.
> Provides a wealth of information on a variety of clinical and management issues, including ethics, supervision, and treatment used in occupational therapy.

Asher, I. E. (1996). *An annotated index of occupational therapy evaluation tools.* Bethesda, MD: American Occupational Therapy Association.
> Provides an annotated list of more than 100 assessments commonly used in occupational therapy. Each assessment summary includes target population, statistical information, and assessment sources.

Bonder, B. R. (2004). *Psychopathology and function.* (3rd ed.). Thorofare, NJ: SLACK Incorporated.
> Major psychiatric disorders are described according to symptomatology, etiology, and prognosis with implications for function and treatment. A description of occupational therapy treatment with reference to *The Practice Framework* is provided.

Borg, B., & Bruce, M. A. (1991). *The group system.* Thorofare, NJ: SLACK Incorporated.
> Provides discussion of the small therapeutic group, its relationship to occupational therapy, and comparison to system theories and group dynamics theories. A major goal of the presenters is to give practical information to group leaders through examples.

Bruce, M. A., & Borg, B. (2002). *Frames of reference in psychosocial occupational therapy.* (3rd ed.). Thorofare, NJ: SLACK Incorporated.
> Six frames of reference in psychiatric occupational therapy are discussed in detail including developmental, cognitive, cognitive behavioral, object relations, behavioral, and occupational behavioral. Additional information on organic mental disorders and the suicidal patient is included.

Christiansen, C. (2004). *Ways of living.* (3rd ed.). Bethesda, MD: American Occupational Therapy Association. Provides detailed analysis of social and physical activities of daily living from basic to community skills.

Christiansen, C., & Baum, C. (1997). *Occupational therapy: Enabling function and well-being.* (2nd ed.). Thorofare, NJ: SLACK Incorporated.
Provides framework of occupational therapy and identifies the links between theory and practice. Discusses reasoning and decision-making processes necessary for competent occupational therapy practice.

Cole, M. (1998). *Group dynamics in occupational therapy.* (2nd ed.). Thorofare, NJ: SLACK Incorporated.
Provides an explanation of the theoretical base of occupational therapy group treatment. Organized as a work book, this book provides guidelines and suggestions for occupational therapists and students to use and implement group process in treatment.

Crepeau, E. B. (2003). *Willard and Spackman's occupational therapy.* (10th ed.). Philadelphia: J. B. Lippincott.
A resource for general professional issues including occupational therapy history, philosophy, occupational science, 11 frames of reference, and practice issues across the lifespan.

Dunn, W. (1991). *Pediatric occupational therapy.* Thorofare, NJ: SLACK Incorporated.
Discusses both service and support models of pediatric occupational therapy referral, screening, assessment, and treatment. Includes family, educators, and medical perspectives. Assessments commonly used are discussed, as well as documentation and marketing.

Dunn, W. (2000). *Best practice occupational therapy.* Thorofare, NJ: SLACK Incorporated.
Theoretical and evidence-based knowledge is presented specific to the treatment of children and families. Worksheets and case studies provide opportunities to apply knowledge.

Fiorentino, M. R. (1972). *Normal and abnormal development.* Springfield, IL: Charles C. Thomas Publishing.
A classic resource on the influence of primitive reflexes on motor development. This text provides an orientation to the developmental motor milestones in the normal child. In addition, examples of abnormal development seen in cerebral palsy are also featured.

Frender, G. (1990). *Learning to learn.* Nashville, TN: Incentives Publications.
A hands-on guide of practical hints, methods, tips, procedures, and tools for learning how to learn. Includes topics such as learning styles, organizational skills, memory, time management, and test-taking skills.

Gilfoyle, E. M., Grady, A. P., & Moore, J. C. (1990). *Children adapt.* Thorofare, NJ: SLACK Incorporated.
The theory of sensorimotor-sensory development is presented with nervous system and spatiotemporal adaptation highlighted. Developmental sequences are used in treatment to gain skilled performance.

Hansen, R., & Atchison, B. (2000). *Conditions in occupational therapy: Effects on occupational performance.* Baltimore: Williams & Wilkins.
Pathophysiology of major conditions most frequently seen in occupational therapy clinics are reviewed. Diagnostic tests, medical management, and occupational performance perspectives are addressed in case study reviews.

Hemphill-Pearson, B. (1999). *Assessment in occupational therapy mental health: An integrative approach.* Thorofare, NJ: SLACK Incorporated.
Provides in-depth discussion on several commonly used assessments in psychiatric occupational therapy, including assessments for independent living skills and work. In addition, a detailed chapter on the interview process is included.

Hinojosa, J., & Kramer, P. (1998). *Evaluation: Obtaining and interpreting data.* Bethesda, MD: American Occupational Therapy Association.

> Evaluation and assessment basics such as psychometric standards and development are addressed. This book looks at standardized and nonstandardized assessments across the specialties.

Jacobs, K. (2004). *Quick reference dictionary for occupational therapy.* (4th ed.). Thorofare, NJ: SLACK Incorporated.

> Provides definitions of occupational therapy terms, concepts, and conditions, as well as informative appendices.

Jacobs, K., & Logigian, M. (1999). *Functions of a manager in occupational therapy.* (3rd ed.). Thorofare, NJ: SLACK Incorporated.

> This text covers a wide variety of management and administrative responsibilities of the OT.

Kaplan, H. I., Sadock, B. J., & Grebb, J. A. (2002). *Synopsis of psychiatry.* (9th ed.). Baltimore: Williams & Wilkins.

> Provides an extensive reference and explanation of the DSM-IV, including all psychiatric classifications from various theoretical models. Clinical explanations and classic treatment are described in detail.

Kaplan, K. L. (1988). *Directive group therapy.* Thorofare, NJ: SLACK Incorporated.

> Provides concepts and practical guidance of this therapy model designed specifically for the person functioning at a minimal level.

Katz, N. (1998). *Cognition and occupation in rehabilitation.* Bethesda, MD: American Occupational Therapy Association.

> Complete coverage of a variety of cognitive issues across the specialties including chronic mental health issues and traumatic brain injury.

Kiernat, J. M. (1991). *Occupational therapy and the older adult: A clinical manual.* Gaithersburg, MD: Aspen Publications.

> This text reviews aging, functional changes, and adaptation of adults over 65 years. Treatment information includes the role of fitness, empowerment, preventing falls, and cognition aspects. Medicare is fully reviewed. Both community and long-term treatment are discussed in detail, including assessment, treatment, and discharge planning.

Law, M. (1998). *Client-centered occupational therapy.* Thorofare, NJ: SLACK Incorporated.

> Explains the models available to center treatment around client's goals. The Canadian Model of Occupational Performance is fully explained.

Leonard, P. C. (2003). *Quick and easy medical terminology.* (4th ed.). Philadelphia: W. B. Saunders Company.

> A self-study test that provides a repetition and quiz format for learning medical terminology.

Levangie, P. (2001). *Joint structure and function: A comprehensive analysis.* (3rd ed.). Philadelphia: F. A. Davis Company.

> Presents basic theory of joint structure and muscle action necessary to understanding both normal and abnormal function. A review of biomechanics is included.

Lewis, S. C. (2003). *Elder care in occupational therapy.* (2nd ed.). Thorofare, NJ: SLACK Incorporated.

> A detailed text on normal development and challenges of aging. Disease processes and treatments are discussed, including discussion on death and dying. Medicare laws, rules, and funding are fully described.

Millen, H. M. (1978). *Body mechanics and safe transfer techniques.* Detroit, MI: Aronsson Printing.

> A practical guide with numerous photographs of proper body mechanics and transfers of patients. Discusses special techniques for heavy transfers and emergency transfers.

Moyers, P. (1999). *Guide to occupational therapy practice.* Bethesda, MD: American Occupational Therapy Association.

> A comprehensive review of the literature that supports the field of occupational therapy. Focus is on basic concepts such as the OT process and referrals for services. Excellent to use when explaining OT to another profession.

National Board for Certification in Occupational Therapy. (Spring, 2004). *Report to the profession.* Gaithersburg, MD: Author.

> Use the NBCOT web site, www.nbcot.org, for up-to-the-minute news and information concerning both the OT and OTA exams.

Reed, K. L. (2003). *Quick reference to occupational therapy.* (2nd ed.). Gaithersburg, MD: Aspen Publications.

> An extensive review of common disorders across the age span and disability practice. Information on the cause, assessment, and treatment is provided in outline format. Precautions and outcomes are described. References and further readings specific to the disorders are provided.

Schkade, J., & McClung, M. (2001). *Occupational adaptation in practice.* Thorofare, NJ: SLACK Incorporated.

> Discusses the role of environment and fit in helping clients form adaptive responses to occupational roles.

Simmons, P. L., & Mullins, L. (1981). *Acute psychiatric care.* Thorofare, NJ: SLACK Incorporated.

> A practical guide to group exercises in daily living skills. Includes suggestions in leisure, assertiveness, employment, money management, and discharge planning.

Sladyk, K. (1997). *OT student primer: A guide to college success.* Thorofare, NJ: SLACK Incorporated.

> Basic OT concepts and techniques are reviewed.

Sladyk, K. (2003). *OT study cards in a box* (2nd ed.). Thorofare, NJ: SLACK Incorporated.

> A deck of index-sized cards that review the major content areas for fieldwork, NBCOT exam, or practice.

Sonbuchner, G. M. (1991). *Finding your best learning styles and study environment.* Rochelle Park, NJ: Peoples Publishing Group.

> A booklet designed to determine one's best learning style. Strategies are presented to enhance particular learning strengths.

Sonbuchner, G. M. (1991). *Time management.* Rochelle Park, NJ: Peoples Publishing Group.

> A booklet presenting basic time management strategies including time-saving tips, making better use of study time, and keeping track of things that need to be done.

Trombly, C., & Radomski, M. (2002). *Occupational therapy for physical dysfunction.* (5th ed.). Baltimore: Williams & Wilkins.

> Principles of practice in adult physical dysfunction are featured. Major diagnostic areas are covered with focus on assessment and treatment. Numerous photographs illustrate basic techniques.

Wilcock, A. (1998). *An occupational perspective of health.* Thorofare, NJ: SLACK Incorporated.

> Examines the relationship of health and occupation by defining and exploring occupation biologically and socially.

Williams, L., Pedretti, L., & Early, M. B. (2001). *Occupational therapy skills for physical dysfunction.* St. Louis, MO: Mosby.

> A basic-level reference for clinicians, this text provides the application techniques for the treatment of adults with acquired physical dysfunction. Occupational therapy evaluation and treatment issues are addressed.

Yalom, I. D. (1985). *The theory and practice of group psychotherapy.* New York: Basic Books.
   Provides a scholarly review of various group therapy models based on recent developments in the field, as well as the author's expertise with clinical syndromes.

Zemke, R., & Clark, F. (1996). *Occupational science: The evolving discipline.* Philadelphia: F.A. Davis Company.
   Provides a model for understanding occupation as a science and art before examining occupational therapy treatment as an end means.

Zoltan, B. (1996). *Vision, perception, and cognition: A manual for the evaluation and treatment of the neurologically impaired adult.* (3rd ed.). Thorofare, NJ: SLACK Incorporated.
   Manual defines and outlines the theoretical basis of visual, perceptual, and cognitive deficits. Evaluation procedures and treatment are also identified.

Appendix B
Helpful Abbreviations

The following is a list of abbreviations you may find helpful. You do not need to commit them to memory for the OT exam, however, a working knowledge of them is useful.

ADA	Americans with Disabilities Act
ADL	activities of daily living
AIDS	acquired immune deficiency syndrome
AOTA	American Occupational Therapy Association
AOTF	American Occupational Therapy Foundation
AROM	active range of motion
CARF	Commission of Accredited Rehabilitation Facilities
COPD	chronic obstructive pulmonary disease
COTE	Comprehensive Occupational Therapy Evaluation
CVA	cerebral vascular accident
DIP	distal interphalangeal
DRG	diagnosis related groups
ECT	electroconvulsive therapy
FOR	frame of reference
HMO	health maintenance organization
JCAHO	Joint Commission on Accreditation of Healthcare Organizations
MCP	metacarpal phalangeal
MET	metabolic equivalents
MMT	manual muscle test
MORE	measurable, observable, realistic, explicit
NBCOT	National Board for Certification in Occupational Therapy

OBRA	Omnibus Budget Reconciliation Act
OSHA	Occupational Safety and Health Administration
OT	occupational therapy, occupational therapist
OTA	occupational therapy assistant
PIP	proximal interphalangeal
POMR	problem-oriented medical record
PRN	whenever necessary
PROM	passive range of motion
ROM	range of motion
SOAP	subjective, objective, assessment, plan
SSI/SSD	Social Security Insurance/Social Security Disability

Appendix C

Authors' Feedback Form

The authors need your help!

As the consumer of this study guide, you have valuable information that you can provide the authors of this book. Please take a few minutes after you are finished studying with this book and tell us what was beneficial about it and what needs improvement. Future occupational therapy students will greatly benefit from your insight.

1. Please list the sections of the book you found helpful.

2. What was the most helpful?

3. Could you briefly tell us why it was the most helpful?

4. Please list the sections of the book you feel need improvement.

5. What was the least helpful?

6. Could you briefly tell us why it was the least helpful?

7. Where or how did you find this book?

8. Do you think this book should be an optional textbook in OT school?

9. Do you think this book should be a required textbook in OT school?

Is there anything else you would like to tell us?
About you:

Your age:

Your gender:

Circle the type of degree you have or will earn:
BA   BS   Post BS Certificate   MA   MS   MOT

Mail the completed form to Karen Sladyk, PhD, OTR/L, FAOTA, in care of SLACK Incorporated, Professional Book Division, 6900 Grove Road, Thorofare, NJ 08086.

Index

WAIT

...There's More!

SLACK Incorporated's Professional Book Division offers a wide selection of products in the field of Occupational Therapy. We are dedicated to providing important works that educate, inform and improve the knowledge of our customers. Don't miss out on our other informative titles that will enhance your collection.

OT Study Cards in a Box, Second Edition
Karen Sladyk, PhD, OTR/L, FAOTA

255 Cards with Carrier, 2003, ISBN 1-55642-620-8, Order #36208, $43.95

OT Study Cards in a Box has been completely revised and updated into a comprehensive second edition perfect for both OT & OTA students and clinicians. The user-friendly format includes tabs located on the side of the cards for easy navigation of the subject areas. Whether a student is preparing for the certification exam or a clinician simply needs a reminder, *OT Study Cards in a Box, Second Edition* provides the facts needed at a moments glance.

Quick Reference Dictionary for Occupational Therapy, Fourth Edition
Karen Jacobs, EdD, OTR/L, CPE, FAOTA and Laela Jacobs, OTR

600 pp., Soft Cover, 2004, ISBN 1-55642-656-9, Order #36569, $26.95

This definitive companion provides quick access to words, their definitions, and important resources used in everyday practice and the classroom. Used by thousands of your peers and colleagues, the *Quick Reference Dictionary for Occupational Therapy, Fourth Edition* is one of a kind and needed by all in the profession.

OT Exam Review Manual, Fourth Edition
Karen Sladyk, PhD, OTR/L, FAOTA; Signian McGeary, MS, OTR/L; Lori S. Gilmore, MS, CSE; and Roseanna Tufano, MFT, OTR/L

224 pp., Soft Cover, 2005, ISBN 1-55642-702-6, Order #37026, $29.95

OT Student Primer: A Guide to College Success
Karen Sladyk, PhD, OTR/L, FAOTA

348 pp., Soft Cover, 1997, ISBN 1-55642-318-7, Order #33187, $32.95

The Successful Occupational Therapy Fieldwork Student
Karen Sladyk, PhD, OTR/L, FAOTA

240 pp., Soft Cover, 2002, ISBN 1-55642-562-7, Order #35627, $35.95

Quick Reference Dictionary for Occupational Therapy for the PDA, Fourth Edition
Karen Jacobs, EdD, OTR/L, CPE, FAOTA and Laela Jacobs, OTR

PDA, 2004, ISBN 1-55642-705-0, Order #37050, $26.95

Quick Reference Neuroscience for Rehabilitation Professionals: The Essential Neurologic Principles Underlying Rehabilitation Practice
Sharon A. Gutman, PhD, OTR

288 pp., Soft Cover, 2001, ISBN 1-55642-463-9, Order #34639, $38.95

Documentation Manual for Writing SOAP Notes in Occupational Therapy
Sherry Borcherding, MA, OTR/L

256 pp., Soft Cover, 2000, ISBN 1-55642-441-8, Order #34418, $29.95

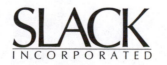